I0791703

TRANSITION BACK TO THE NATURAL HUMAN
DIET WITH EASE

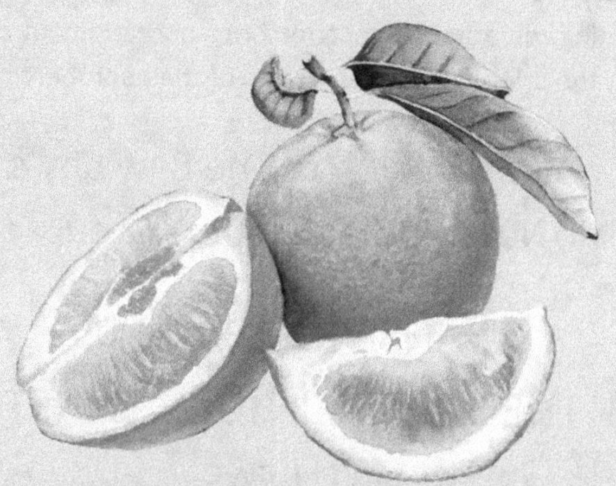

THE NATURAL HUMAN DIET

Quick Start Guide

BY LAUREN WHITEMAN, MARIA MANAZZA, AND NAT FARRIS

TheRawKey.com & AppleDiaries.com

The Natural Human Diet Quick Start Guide

A Companion to The Raw Key's
Natural Diet Support Group

TRANSITION BACK TO
THE NATURAL HUMAN DIET
WITH EASE

Grocery Lists, Meal Plans, and Recipes to support your transition.

By Lauren Whiteman, Maria Manazza and Nat Farris

Updated to include even more information on how to transition to the natural human diet, with additional meal plans, and recipes, including Summer Party Recipes and Camping Favorites, information about our monthly support group, and testimonials from group members.

Edited and published with BookPrints
Printed by kdp.amazon.com
Revision 2.22, February 2025

022625.pb.R2.22

The Natural Human Diet Quick Start Guide
Table of Contents

The Natural Human Diet Quick Start Guide
Table of Contents

The Natural Human Diet Quick Start Guide
Table of Contents

Table of Contents

The Natural Human Diet Quick Start Guide
Table of Contents

The Natural Human Diet
Introduction
How to Use this Guide

Welcome to TheRawKey.com's Natural Diet Support Group! This Quick Start Guide was created to inspire you and give you guidance, support, and clarity as you move towards the natural human diet and healing, and to accompany and supplement the monthly online support group, hosted by Lauren Whiteman, Maria Manazza and Nat Farris.

Meal Plan Options We have included weekly meal plans for those who are striving for fully raw and hygienic (The Natural Human Diet), another plan for those who are looking to stay raw but are not quite ready for fully hygienic (Transitional Raw), and other options for those who still need some cooked foods to keep them on track (Transitional with Cooked Foods). Following the meal plans is optional, and you can stick strictly to one category or mix things up.

Recipes A full range of recipes are included for getting started, for transitioning diet choices and for fully raw / hygienic options, supporting the three Meal Plan Options. Recipes are included for juices and smoothies, breakfast items, salads and dressings, soups, snacks, appetizers and entrees. There are even hygienic recipes for cheeses, butters, and jams, dips and spreads. A separate Holiday Guide includes three Holiday Menus and corresponding recipe options. After that we have added some fun and tasty Summer Recipes and Camping Favorites.

Goals Your immediate goal is to find what works for you, where you are right now. Examine your current habits and trends, and identify your best options for making successful changes. Small changes have cascading effects. The meal plans and recipes in this guide can be helpful in setting your own wellness goals, whether you follow a seven-day meal plan, change your breakfast / lunch, or make adjustments a few days a week to get started. We recommend you go at your own pace and go with what works for you.

Our Goals are to present the tenets of Natural Hygiene and provide guidance and support to those who strive to transition to a healthier lifestyle, so that they can make informed choices. No one is expected to strictly adhere to hygienic foods and there is no judgment. We teach the ideals of natural hygiene, but we recognize that everyone is in a different place and has different wellness goals, short and long term.

Whatever your goals are, you can use the Meal Plans provided, or modify them to your own tastes. You can test out the recipes and use them as inspiration to invent your own. Or you can opt to eat simply, which is the most ideal option and the ultimate end goal.

What is Hygienic?

A hygienic diet, or the natural human diet, is based upon the science of natural hygiene. Natural hygiene is a body of scientific knowledge that shows us how disease is created and reversed, and how to encourage the condition of good health to prevent and reverse disease. Natural hygiene also teaches us how the body self-cleans and self-repairs, and what the natural foods of mankind are which support our health. The science of natural hygiene identifies our most ideal foods, which cause no harm and allow the body to operate under normal parameters and function properly and optimally. This knowledge base also tells us what substances are harmful or irritating to the body, thus creating a burden on bodily functions.

In terms of eating hygienically this means eating as simply as possible of the most ideal foods possible; a diet that is predominantly fruits and lettuce greens, with small amounts of nuts, seeds and tender vegetables. It also means avoiding all substances that are irritating or harmful to the body, which include herbs, spices, salt, spicy peppers, black pepper, garlic, onions, ginger, turmeric and other irritants.

Hygiene

'hī-jēn

noun.

The science that deals with the promotion and preservation of health.

What is Transitional?

Transitional describes the gap between how people commonly eat today (cooked foods, meat, dairy, eggs, lots of spices, salt and other harmful irritants) and an ideal health creating diet. We recognize that it is very difficult for most people to make large changes to the diet they have been eating their entire lives; we present ways to make gradual improvements, step by step, to allow for a slow transition and retraining of habits.

With this guide we seek to bridge the gap, by including both the fully hygienic recipes and meal plans as well as transitional plans and recipes which include some cooked foods or some spices, herbs and other substances (marked in recipes as * for "not hygienic") typically used in cooked meals, to replicate familiar flavors, while moving gradually to fully raw. Even if you are not ready for raw foods, we encourage you to take a look at the meal plans and recipes for those sections to see what is ahead for you.

There is no set schedule for transitioning to a hygienic diet. Each journey to this point has been unique, and the path forward is different for each of us. With each small step that you take, you will learn to listen to your body, and determine what works best for you.

If you aren't ready to make big changes or follow a meal plan, you can start with: first meal fruit, second meal salad, and third meal whatever you would usually eat. A small next step would be to replace the third meal with a healthier, cooked or steamed meal. After this, you might switch to a fruit meal, fruit meal, salad meal pattern. As far as what to eliminate, we generally recommend avoiding dairy, wheat and ultra processed foods, followed by meat and spices. Over time it gets much easier and this is generally a decent plan for starting the transition.

During this transition, if you're getting 10-15 clean meals per week, and having some less than ideal foods several times per week, that's a great start. Over time you'll see positive results and you'll also have bigger reactions to the less ideal foods; it gets easier to make the necessary changes.

What Is The Natural Human Diet?

The natural human diet is based on the principles of terrain theory, and models lifestyle choices that follow these health promoting principles. A healthy terrain is best maintained by consuming foods which we are naturally and ideally suited for, creating or adding little burden to bodily functions and systems, and allowing one to thrive. When our terrain becomes burdened with waste from non-ideal food choices, the bacteria that are always present in our body expand their populations to clean the terrain in a constant effort to return the body to normal and natural functions. If we continue to feed the body unsuitable materials, the burden grows and the body must create expulsion symptoms to rid itself of waste. These cleaning symptoms such as cold and flu healing events, fevers and rashes are labeled as diseases and infections in the allopathic medical world. These body processes actually keep our waste levels in check and keep us from moving into a state of chronic disease. When we return to the natural diet our body goes through a period of

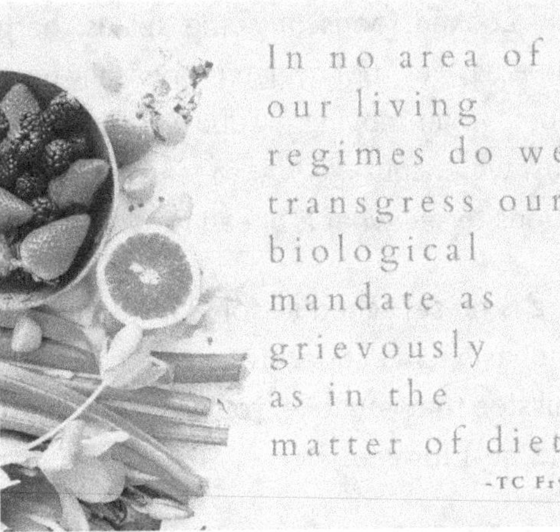

cleansing, ridding itself of the excess waste which has built up over the years and decades of wrong eating; after this has completed the body is returned to a state of pristine health. Pristine health is maintained from this point forward as long as we continue to properly feed our body. If we return to our old habits of eating cooked and other unsuitable foods, disease conditions will also return.

The natural human diet consists of the foods which are most suited to our anatomy and physiology. *Fruits are the predominant food of mankind.* Fruits should make up roughly 50% of our diet by volume for optimal health. The natural human diet also includes sweet tender leafy greens, tender vegetables, nuts and seeds. Leafy greens should be the largest portion of these four items with small quantities of nuts, seeds and vegetables rounding out the diet.

The ideal way to eat the natural diet would be two meals per day, one fruit meal and one salad meal. A salad meal includes a head of lettuce, savory fruits (like tomatoes, cucumbers and zucchini), tender vegetables, and nuts or seeds as desired. Other options include eating one meal a day of fruits mixed with greens, or three meals a day, one fruit, one salad, one nuts/seeds, or two fruit meals and one salad.

It takes some time transitioning from a SAD (Standard American Diet) or cooked foods diet to eating one or two meals per day. It's perfectly fine to start out eating 4 or 5 meals or snacks throughout the day as you first start to move away from cooked foods. Over time as your body rebuilds its store of nutrients and repairs damage you will naturally drift towards fewer meals, less food and simpler meals.

How Is The Natural Human Diet Determined?

Every animal on our planet is capable of eating a certain narrow set of foods. It is understood that the foods most easily accessible and readily available for any particular organism in their natural environment are in fact the foods that incur the smallest possible burden on the organism. Take for example the sea otter. While many of them learn to smash rocks against clam shells to break them open, this is a process that costs more energy than it produces. The sea otter's natural food source then is not clams, but the small fish that occupy the same waters as the otters, and of which they can easily obtain nutrition without over-exerting themselves.

Humans are in the anatomical classification of frugivore – an animal which feeds primarily on fruits, though many pretend to be omnivore – eating both plants and meat. Technically, frugivore is a subcategory of herbivore, which broadly means "plant eater." There are other types of herbivores such as granivores which are mostly rodents, and ruminant herbivores like cows, horses and sheep. Each category has different anatomy and physiology which is designed to acquire, digest and metabolize their ideal foods. Our ideal diet as frugivores, which suits all of our needs without overworking the body's metabolism, consists of fruits and tender greens, with some tender vegetables, nuts, and seeds. Frugivore is a scientific classification which is assigned to the species, based on physical characteristics and observation of behavior and environment. Fruitarian is a dietary choice, like vegetarian, vegan, pescatarian, and other specific eating styles.

Fruits and leafy greens provide everything that humans and all frugivore species require to survive and thrive. Raw whole fruits contain protein in the form of usable amino acids. Fruits also contain small amounts of fats in the form of fatty acids, as well as vitamins (coenzymes), minerals, various trace elements, and most importantly sugar and water, in the form that your body can utilize readily.

The human body runs on carbohydrates, which are also known as sugars. Sugar is the fuel for every one of our hundred trillion cells. However, it is important to make the distinction between simple sugars versus complex sugars and whole foods versus refined foods. Fructose is a simple sugar found in fruits on which we can thrive. Complex sugars, such as glucose, and starches, are less ideal. Artificial sweeteners are not at all suitable. Refined and fractionated foods like white sugar are detrimental and steal nutrients from the body, leaving us damaged and deficient. Fruits in their whole form provide us with the correct type of sugar to fuel every cell in our body and replenish our body's water and nutrient stores.

> "The natural food of man, judging from his structure, appears to consist principally of the fruits, roots, and other succulent parts of vegetables. His hands afford every facility for gathering them; his short but moderately strong jaws on the other hand, and his canines being equal only in length to the other teeth, together with his tuberculated molars on the other, would scarcely permit him either to masticate herbage, or to devour flesh, were these condiments not previously prepared by cooking."
>
> GEORGES CUVIER

In addition to the necessary and proper sugar, the water found in fruit is essential and provides the best hydration for the human body. However, the water found in fruits is not enough for proper hydration and healing.

For most people who have been raised eating a typical SAD, drinking adequate amounts of water is an essential part of the transition to healing and wellness. In short, we recommend working up to a minimum of one gallon of water per day if you are eating fully raw and 2-3 gallons if you are eating cooked foods. Cooked foods significantly dehydrate the body so it is important to drink extra water to account for this dehydration in order to maintain normal eliminations and cellular hydration. We also recommend distilled water as the preferred source, if you cannot get distilled then choose the available water source with the least amount of inorganic minerals (or TDS – Total Dissolved Solids, which can be measured with a water meter.)

It's okay if one gallon of water seems overwhelming when you start. Just work up to it gradually. Most people find that when they set the intention and know their goal that they are able to increase their water consumption up to one gallon within 3-4 weeks.

How Do We Know What Our Natural Foods Are?

Fruit grows abundantly in what would be our natural, unadulterated habitat, fruit creates the least burden because it is a match for our anatomy and physiology.

Our Senses Our senses are ideally suited for fruit-finding and eating! For example, we *see* in vivid colors, while carnivores and omnivores have a limited color range. Human sight is anatomically designed to be attracted to the bright, pleasing colors of ripe fruit.

We have long slender fingers with a delicate sense of *touch* to reach into trees and bushes and find the delicate fruits and pluck them from the tree. Our hands are perfectly designed to grasp and pluck both large fruits and small berries.

We have a weak sense of *smell* because fruits have strong, pungent, pleasing aromas when they are ripe so we do not need to have a strong sense of smell. Conversely, carnivores and omnivores have a strong sense of smell because prey foods do not have strong smells. Humans can only smell rotting animal carcasses and their smell is repulsive to us. A dog on the other hand can smell a prey animal that walked a path an hour ago and follow its scent for miles.

Humans have a "sweet tooth." Our *taste* buds are tuned to allow us to sense when our natural food is ripe and ready to be eaten as well as to avoid poisons. Bitter tastes tell us that the fruit is unripe or a food is toxic. Sour tells us the fruit is overripe, rotting, and no longer suitable. Some fruits contain a little bit of salty flavor, but overly salty foods burn and cause discomfort to our senses. Touching a spoonful of salt to our tongue results in clear discomfort. Spicy tastes burn our tongue, make us sweat, and our nose runs to warn us that it is toxic. But sweet tastes tell us that our natural food is perfectly ripe and ready to provide us with the essential sugars our body needs to run every cell.

Taste buds are not for emotional highs. They are for survival. They are the messages which tell us what is food and what is poison and when our foods are ready to be eaten.

We crave sugary desserts after heavy meals because our cells are desperately seeking energy. Sugar is what our body converts into ATP (adenosine triphosphate), which is energy, this process is called glycolysis. Every cell in our body, from our brain to the tips of our toes uses sugar to run itself. When we properly feed our body on fruits and provide adequate amounts of sugar to fuel all of our cells, those intense cravings for ice cream, cakes and cookies disappear.

We are attracted to the sweet taste and vibrant colors of fruits. They appeal to us and delight our senses. When we look upon a bowl of apples our mouth waters, when we look upon a baby rabbit our thoughts are turned to protection and care, not to mouthwatering. The sight and smell of blood and gore repulses us. We cook animal tissues and coat them in fruit-based sauces (orange sauce, barbeque sauce, ketchup) or stimulants (pepper, cumin, paprika, and other spices or herbs) to make them palatable to our senses. We are not naturally attracted to the flavors of raw unadulterated animal tissues. We do not salivate at the sight of blood, we are repulsed by it. We do not relish eating the intestines or bones or organs of a warm body. But all carnivores and omnivores do.

Anatomy All carnivores and omnivores eat the bones, feet, fur, and feathers of their prey, and have the natural capabilities to do so, because these are all essential parts of their diet. Did you know you can kill a dog by feeding them meat without bone? But they can survive and thrive on bones with just tiny meat scraps attached. Humans *cannot properly digest* bones, feet, fur or feathers, or raw flesh and find it unappealing to crunch down on a bone. Dogs and cats on the other hand will chew on bones with great excitement and get mental satisfaction from this activity.

Carnivores and omnivores all have sharp fangs and claws to facilitate ripping through the skin and breaking through the skull bones of their prey. Humans have *weak nails* perfect for scoring the skin of fruit but useless for ripping the flesh off of a chicken or a cow. Humans have weak *teeth and incisors* for breaking the skin of an apple or a pear and taking chunks out of fruits. Chewing on bones would damage and break our delicate teeth. And though we do have teeth that are frequently confused for canines, our incisors, they're not sharp like a cats'. They're not meant to break the skin and draw blood, whereas a kitten can do this effortlessly. They are instead, perfect for breaking the skin of fruits and for opening the shells of nuts.

These are just a few of the anatomical features and characteristics of humans which determine our natural diet of juicy, water-rich, easy-to-digest, sugar-filled fruits.

Getting Started

Now that you know what the natural diet is and how it was determined, the next step is to start transitioning back to your natural diet, to recover your health and return your body to the pristine clean terrain that you deserve.

No one can make all of the necessary changes all at once, whether it is adding new foods, or eliminating unwanted foods. Here are some guidelines for what to eliminate first, based on common goals:

If your goal is to lose weight: Cut out dairy, alcohol and salt first.

If your goal is to get out of pain: Cut out dairy, wheat, spices, salt and spicy peppers first.

If your goal is to improve neurological issues: Cut out food coloring, spices, wheat and refined flours, refined sugar and dairy first.

Whether you use one of these goals as a starting point or not, take a look in your pantry and fridge and see what your biggest offenders are right now, which can you stop buying, which can you throw in the trash. Start with whatever feels easiest to release and kick that habit to the curb this week. Next week pick another.

You deserve to be happy. You deserve to be healthy. You deserve to wake each day in a body that is free from pain. You deserve to wake every day with abundant energy and an excitement to seize the day. The choice is yours to make. Eat fruit and be well, or eat cooked foods and slowly degenerate. Choose health and join us today by making a better choice one meal at a time.

Below you will find a printable grocery list to start filling your home with fresh, ripe, delicious fruits and greens. We recommend buying between 3-5 pounds of fruits and greens per person per day. Check the sale flyers, what is on sale is usually what is ripe and in season, which is why the store has a lot of it and is putting it on sale. Fill up your cart with all your favorites. Reviewing the meal plans may also help with your shopping list. Remember to grab at least one head of lettuce per person per day – eating your greens is essential! If you are not yet a big fan of salads feel free to blend those leafy greens into green smoothies. Eventually you will start to crave the salads. Especially with the help of some wonderful simple salad dressings.

Beyond the grocery list, you will find food combining information and chart, meal plans and recipes. At the end of the guide we have a holiday section with menus of different meal plans for your party, and the recipes to go along with each of them. We have updated the Guide to include Hot Beverage alternatives, Summer

Party Recipes and Camping Favorites. We hope you will enjoy trying some of these fun and tasty new recipes. We also added a section for testimonials and success stories from members of our monthly support group.

Happy reading and eating!

Lauren, Maria and Nat

TheRawKey.com

AppleDiaries.com

THE NATURAL HUMAN DIET

GROCERY LIST

Fruits
____Apples
____Pears
____Bananas
____Strawberries
____Blueberries
____Raspberries
____Blackberries
____Oranges
____Grapefruit
____Lemons
____Limes
____Clementine
____Mangos
____Papaya
____Kiwi
____Pineapple
____Coconut (mature)
____Thai Young Coconut
____Cherries
____Peaches
____Nectarines
____Watermelons
____Cantaloupes
____Honeydew Melons
____Papayas
____Grapes
____
____
____

Savory Fruits/Vegetables
____Avocado
____Cucumber
____Romaine Lettuce
____Tomato
____Iceberg Lettuce
____Bibb Lettuce
____Green Leaf Lettuce
____Red Leaf Lettuce
____Celery
____Bell Pepper
____Zucchini
____Yellow Squash
____Mushrooms
____Cabbage
____Kale/Baby Kale
____Spinach/Baby Spinach
____Mixed Greens
____Asparagus
____Corn
____Peas
____Green Beans
____Cauliflower
____Collard Greens
____Carrots
____Snap Peas
____
____
____

Frozen Fruits
____Blueberries
____Mangos
____Dark Sweet Cherries
____Pineapple
____Strawberries
____Mixed Berries
____Dragon Fruit
____Acai
____Raspberries
____Peaches
____Bananas
____
____

Pantry Items
____Chia Seeds
____Flax Seeds
____Hemp Seeds
____Sesame Seeds
____Sunflower Seeds
____Pumpkin Seeds
____Raw Cashews
____Raw Almonds
____Raw Pecans
____Raw Walnuts
____Unsulfured Dried Fruits
____Brazil Nuts
____Hazelnuts
____

Food Combining

We derive no value from foods that are not digested. Fermenting or putrefying food in the digestive tract not only wastes the food itself but is injurious to the body. Undigested fruit ferments creating alcohol to poison the body. Far worse, the putrefaction process of meat releases ammonia. Proper food combining is important because it assures better nutrition as a consequence of better digestion and avoidance of poisoning.

Foods as we eat them, in the form of carbohydrates, proteins, and fats are not usable by the body, as-is. They must undergo a series of disintegrating, refining, and standardizing processes which we call digestion. Digestion is both a physical process and a chemical process. The body creates enzymes to break apart the larger elements of our foods into smaller usable elements that can pass into the bloodstream. Each enzyme is specific in its action. The enzyme that acts upon carbohydrates does not and cannot act upon proteins, salts, or fats. Even down to more specifics, the enzyme that breaks down maltose is not capable of breaking down lactose, despite both being sugars (carbohydrates). Each enzyme has specific conditions required to work adequately and the conditions of an enzyme are often contrary to that of another, so much so as to halt the digestion of one type of substance when the conditions are wrong for that substance.

Most of the time, the ingestion of mixed meals leads to improper digestion, lack of absorption, fermentation, and putrefaction, all of which contribute negatively to our health.

If we are to eat mixed meals, then care should be taken as often as possible to maximize the combinations which digest suitably in each other's presence, and minimize those combinations which digest poorly together.

Dr. Shelton's original 9 food combining rules:

1. Never eat carbohydrate foods and acid foods at the same meal.

2. Never eat a concentrated protein and a concentrated carbohydrate at the same meal.

3. Never consume two concentrated proteins at the same meal.

4. Do not consume fats with proteins.

5. Do not eat acidic fruits with proteins.

6. Do not consume starches and sugars together.

7. Eat but one concentrated starch at a meal.

8. Do not consume melons with any other foods.

9. Milk is best taken alone or let alone.

Simplified Version

1. Eat melons alone or leave them alone

2. Greens are neutral and pair well with almost everything

3. Don't mix sweet fruits with acidic fruits

4. Don't mix fats with sweet fruits

These abridged rules are not perfect, but if we are eating mostly simple meals, then the small number of combined meals we have are not a huge burden. If you get the food combined a little wrong your body will tell you with gas, bloating, or discomfort, and next time you simply don't make that combination again.

FOOD COMBINING

Melons

Watermelon Cantaloupe   Honeydew
Canary   Crenshaw   Casaba

Eat melons alone or with other melons. Melons digest rapidly and will ferment if they move too slowly. Avoid eating melons too soon after a slow-digesting meal, or when digestion is sluggish.

Sweet Fruits

Bananas
Dates
Grapes
Dried Fruits
Persimmons
Papaya

Sub-Acid Fruits

Figs   Apples (sweet)
Apricots   Raspberries
Cherries   Peach
Mangos   Blueberries
Pears   Plums
Kiwis

Acid Fruits

Pineapple
Tangerines
Strawberries
Oranges
Blackberries
Tomatoes
Gooseberries

Sweet can pair with sub-acid. Sub-acid can pair with acid.
Acid does not pair with sweet. All three can pair with lettuce greens.
Fats pair well with savory and greens but not with sweet, acid, and sub-acid.
Starches pair with savory and green vegetables, but not with acid, sweet or protein.

Savory Fruits

Zucchini
Summer Squash
Bell Peppers
Cucumbers

Fats/ Proteins

Seeds
Nuts
Avocado
Nut Butters
Coconut

Greens, Vegetables & Starches

Lettuces   Carrots*
Green Beans   Collard Greens**
Fresh Peas   Brussels Sprouts**
Celery   Kale**
Broccoli **   Cabbage**
Cauliflower**   Spinach
                Corn

*Root vegetables are less ideal due to high starch content and low digestibility
**Dark Leafy greens and cruciferous vegetables contain mild irritants - consume them less often
Corn is considered a sweet fruit when young and tender, a starch as it ages. Best eaten alone or with salad greens and savory fruits.
Simple meals are always the preference.
Ideal eating window is 12pm to 8pm, this is when digestion is most optimal.

Learn more about The Natural Human Diet at TheRawKey.com

* This is meant to be a cheat sheet / rough guide – not all combining rules are included *

Notes on Meal Plans and Recipes

Meal Plan Options and Recipes We have included two meal plans for Fully Raw and Hygienic – one with two meals and a snack, and another with three meals and two snacks. We recognize that even if you have chosen a raw meal plan, you may still need to transition over time to eating fewer meals throughout the day. There is one meal plan for Transitional Raw, and there are two options for Transitional with Cooked foods: Three meals with one or two snacks and a "Raw 'Til Dinner" plan. You can stick to one meal plan for the entire week, or mix things up as you see fit.

Capitalized items on a meal plan indicate a Recipe. All recipes are to be viewed as a rough guide and to be used for inspiration to make your own creations. They can be tweaked and modified to suit your own tastes and purposes. Many of the recipes are meant for transitional purposes – as a way to step into the fully raw lifestyle, and include non-ideal ingredients and methods. Therefore not all recipes are completely hygienic – * next to an ingredient indicates "not hygienic" – feel free to exclude or substitute with another choice.

Bragg Liquid Aminos (Braggs) is a product included in some recipes, to add flavor for transitional foods and meals. It is made from soybeans, and often used as a substitute for soy sauce. They also make a coconut aminos product (no soybeans) which could be used interchangeably in the recipes. If you prefer you can substitute tamari, which is a fermented by-product of miso production with a similar savory flavor as Braggs, but stronger and with less sodium. When using tamari instead of Braggs cut the amount by half and adjust to taste. Neither product is considered hygienic.

A Note about Calories We have noted an estimated caloric value of all of our recipes and meal plans. These values are rounded and may not be entirely consistent. The purpose of displaying the calorie values is to allow people to get a rough idea of the number of calories in the listed food item, so we tried to make this simple by using round numbers. Furthermore, we have taken a rough estimate of the total caloric value of an entire recipe and then tried to distribute it into servings. For juices, we have estimated that juice contains approximately 80% of the caloric value of the whole food.

It should be emphasized that these are rough estimates. Not only is it true that no two peppers or figs or apples are the same, but it is also true that calories are only one facet of the story of nutrition of food. We recommend being aware of caloric value without obsession.

Cronometer.com was used to get values for the food, and it is recommended to use this service occasionally to ensure you are eating roughly enough quantity of food. It can be common for people to under eat when swapping to a more raw and natural diet because raw and unprocessed foods are much less dense than cooked foods, so we generally need a greater volume of food and this can be difficult to adjust to.

Culinary Herbs and Spices While culinary herbs and spices are not hygienic and would never be recommended, we understand that many people may prefer to add them to recipes in the short term to get accustomed to eating this way. As such we have indicated in many recipes when certain herbs or spices might be complementary. As always, what you decide to prepare and eat is at your discretion.

Meal Plans

Fully Raw and Hygienic – The Natural Human Diet

Ideally, a hygienic meal plan would start no earlier than Noon, with the last meal completed before 8 pm, to match the natural digestive phase.

2 Meals Per Day + Snack – 1700-2400 calories

See Recipes sections for combined foods (Capitalized Items).
Drink water upon waking until first meal / snack.

Day 1 – 2000 calories

Break Fast 12 Noon – 625 calories

Snack 3pm – 850 calories

Late Afternoon Meal 6 pm – 525 calories

2 pounds grapes

8 medium bananas

Spinach Salad with Sweet Tomato Dressing

Day 2 –1885 calories

Break Fast 12 Noon – 1050 calories

Snack 3pm – 400 calories

Late Afternoon Meal 6 pm – 435 calories

10 medium bananas

6 medjool dates

Tomato, Cucumber, and Zucchini Salad with Tomato Mango Dressing

Day 3 – 1980 calories

Break Fast 12 Noon – 550 calories

Afternoon Meal 4 pm – 1145 calories

4 pounds of watermelon

Banana Tacos with dates (8 bananas + 4 medjool dates + 1 head of romaine lettuce)

Snack 7 pm – 285 calories

1 pound cherries

Day 4 – 1700 calories
Break Fast 12 Noon – 725 calories
Snack 3 pm – 550 calories
Late Afternoon Meal 6pm – 425 calories

3-pound bag of mandarin oranges
10 dried smyrna figs
Zoodles with Creamy Tomato
Dressing (4 medium zucchini +
Full Dressing Recipe)

Day 5 – 1770 calories
Break Fast 12 Noon – 570 calories
Snack 3 pm – 630 calories
Late Afternoon Meal 6 pm – 570 calories

6 medium apples
6 medium bananas
Simple Salad with Mango Dressing

Day 6 – 2400 calories
Break Fast 12 Noon – 600 calories
Snack 3 pm – 550 calories

Late Afternoon Meal 6 pm – 1250 calories

7 large oranges
3 medium apples with Date
Caramel (4 medjool dates + 2
tbsp water blended)
10 Mixed Berry Tacos

Day 7 – 2040 calories
Break Fast 12 Noon – 640 calories

Afternoon Meal 4pm – 860 calories

Snack 7 pm – 540 calories

2 pints blueberries, 4 medium
bananas
6 ears of sweet corn
Simple Salad with Sweet Tomato
Dressing
2 medium zucchini, sliced
1 medium cucumber, sliced
Red Pepper Cashew Cheese (½
portion of Recipe)

Fully Raw and Hygienic – The Natural Human Diet

Ideally, a hygienic meal plan would start no earlier than Noon, with the last meal completed before 8 pm, to match the natural digestive phase.

3 Meals + 2 Snacks Per Day – 1700-2100 calories

See Recipes sections for combined foods (Capitalized Items).
Drink water upon waking until first meal / snack.

Day 1 – 1765 calories

Snack 9am – 270 calories — Date Beverage or other Hot Beverage

Meal 12pm – 315 calories — 1 pound of grapes
Meal 2pm – 525 calories — 5 medium bananas
Snack 5pm – 315 calories — 1 cup dried apricots
Meal 7pm – 340 calories — Simple Avocado Salad

Day 2 – 1785 calories

Meal 9am – 315 calories — 1 pound of grapes
Meal 12pm – 285 calories — 1 pound of cherries
Meal 2pm – 735 calories — 7 bananas
Snack 5pm – 270 calories — Date Beverage or other Hot Beverage

Snack 7pm – 180 calories — ¼ cup cashews

Day 3 – 1980 calories

Meal 9am – 315 calories — 1 pound of grapes
Snack 12pm – 550 calories — 10 dried smyrna figs
Meal 2pm – 255 calories — 5 peaches
Meal 5pm – 530 calories — Simple Salad Romaine
Snack 7pm – 330 calories — 5 medjool dates

Day 4 – 1895 calories
Meal 9am – 525 calories
Meal 12pm – 315 calories
Snack 2pm – 435 calories
Meal 5pm – 440 calories

Snack 7pm – 180 calories

5 medium bananas
1 pound of grapes
1 cup raisins
Simple Salad with Sweet Red
  Pepper Dressing
¼ cup cashews

Day 5 – 2095 calories
Meal 9am – 285 calories
Meal 12pm – 315 calories
Snack 2pm – 315 calories
Meal 5pm – 630 calories
Snack 7pm – 550 calories

1 pound of cherries
1 pound of grapes
1 cup dried apricots
6 bananas
10 dried smyrna figs

Day 6 – 1985 calories
Snack 9am – 270 calories

Snack 12pm – 660 calories
Meal 2pm – 315 calories
Meal 5pm – 550 calories
Snack 7pm – 190 calories

Date Beverage or other Hot
  Beverage
6 dried smyrna figs
1 pound of grapes
10 Banana Tacos
¼ cup walnuts

Day 7 – 1875 calories
Snack 9am – 270 calories

Snack 12pm – 435 calories
Meal 2pm – 285 calories
Meal 5pm – 335 calories

Snack 7pm – 550 calories

Date Beverage or other Hot
  Beverage
1 cup raisins
1 pound of cherries
Zucchini Noodle Salad with Sweet
  Tomato Dressing
10 dried smyrna figs

Transitional Raw 1600-2400 calories

Higher protein and fat. More smoothies and juices.
May not follow best food combining practices.
See Recipes sections for combined foods (Capitalized Items).
Drink water upon waking until first meal / snack.

Day 1 – 1780 calories

Break Fast – 630 calories

Afternoon Meal – 530 calories

Snack – 220 calories

Evening Meal – 400 calories

Banana Mylk

Classic Tomato Soup

4 dried smyrna figs

Classic Salad

Day 2 – 2090 calories

Break Fast – 540 calories

Afternoon Meal – 630 calories

Snack – 190 calories

Evening Meal – 730 calories

3 Just Bananas Pancakes

6 bananas

¼ cup pecans

Kale Salad with Sweet Orange
  Dressing

Day 3 – 2370 calories

Break Fast – 615 calories

Afternoon Meal – 415 calories

Snack – 1040 calories

Evening Meal – 300 calories

Cherry Smoothie

Kale & Brussels Sprout Salad with
  Lemon Mustard Dressing

Apples with Date Caramel

Collard Wraps

Day 4 – 1965 calories

Break Fast – 345 calories

Afternoon Meal – 400 calories

Snack – 720 calories

Evening Meal – 500 calories

Raw Oatmeal

Veggie Sandwiches

3 pound bag of mandarins

Raw Tacos – using Hygienic Taco
   Filling

Day 5 – 1790 calories

Break Fast – 240 calories

Morning Snack – 525 calories

Afternoon Meal – 490 calories

Snack – 160 calories

Evening Meal – 375 calories

Watermelon Juice

5 medium bananas

Pea Soup

2 tablespoons Raw Peanut Butter

Coodles with Avocado Sauce

Day 6 – 1900 calories

Break Fast – 315 calories

Morning Snack – 430 calories

Afternoon Meal – 275 calories

Snack – 560 calories

Evening Meal – 320 calories

Ultimate Refresher

1 cup raisins

Veggie Burger

2 zucchini and 2 cucumbers sliced
   with Asparagus Dip (half recipe)

Raw Plant-Based Sushi

Day 7 – 1690 calories

Break Fast – 380 calories

Morning Snack – 390 calories

Afternoon Meal – calories 300

Snack – 270 calories

Evening Meal – 350 calories

4 medium apples

Raw Bagel with Cream "Cheese"

Creamy Red Bell Pepper Soup

5 stalks celery sticks with 3 tbsp
   Peanut Butter or other nut
   butter

Raw Fajitas

Transitional with Cooked Foods

3 Meals and 1 or 2 Snacks Per Day – 1700-2600 calories
See Recipes sections for combined foods (Capitalized Items).
Drink water upon waking until first meal / snack.

Day 1 – 1835 calories

Breakfast – 520 calories	Strawberry Banana Smoothie
Morning Snack – 300 calories	5 medjool dates
Lunch – 395 calories	Simple Salad w/ Sunflower Seed Dressing
Dinner – 160 calories	Lentil Soup – 4 servings
Snack – 460 calories	3 medium apples with ¼ cup Cashew Butter

Day 2 – 2080 calories

Breakfast – 630 calories	6 bananas
Lunch – 400 calories	Veggie Sandwiches
Dinner – 500 calories	half recipe of Red Lentil Flatbread with 3-4 cups mixed vegetables
Snack – 550 calories	Hummus with Zucchini Chips (raw or dehydrated)

Day 3 – 1960 calories

Breakfast – 540 calories	Orange Juice
Morning Snack – 280 calories	3 medium apples
Lunch – 260 calories	Raw Asparagus Soup
Dinner – 600 calories	Zoodles with Marinara
Snack – 280 calories	No Oil "Fries" 2 Potatoes

Day 4 – 2240 calories
Breakfast – 315 calories
Morning Snack – 300 calories
Lunch – 415 calories

Dinner – 635 calories

Snack – 575 calories

1 pound grapes
Raw Cinnamon Rolls, 2 Rolls
Kale & Brussels Sprout Salad with
  Lemon Mustard Dressing
Black Bean Soup and Simple Salad
  with Sweet Tomato Dressing
Banana Nice Cream with Raw
  Fudge Brownies

Day 5 – 2575 calories
Breakfast – 1040 calories
Lunch – 545 calories

Dinner – 600 calories

Snack – 390 calories

4-6 Apples with Date Caramel
Coodles with Mango Tomato
  Sauce
Classic Salad with your choice of
  dressing
Raw Bagel with Cream "Cheese"

Day 6 – 2170 calories
Breakfast – 840 calories
Lunch – 550 calories
Dinner – 320 calories
Snack – 460 calories

4 bananas with Date Caramel
Creamy Tomato Soup
Raw Plant-Based Sushi
1 zucchini and 1 cucumber sliced
  with half recipe of Red Pepper
  Cashew Cheese

Day 7 – 1765 calories
Breakfast – 540 calories
Lunch – 670 calories
Dinner – 255 calories

Snack – 300 calories

32 oz orange juice (8-12 oranges)
Corn Soup
Tomato Vegetable Soup with
  baked sweet potato
Blueberry Pie

Transitional with Cooked Foods

Raw 'Til Dinner – 1700-2100 calories

See Recipes sections for combined foods (Capitalized Items).
Drink water upon waking until first meal / snack.

Day 1 – 2115 calories

9am – 270 calories	Date Beverage or other Hot Beverage
12pm – 420 calories	4 medium bananas
2pm – 160 calories	½ cup dried apricots
5pm – 285 calories	1 pound cherries
7pm – 980 calories	Quinoa and Lentil Salad with Sunflower Seed Dressing

Day 2 – 2035 calories

9am – 315 calories	1 pound of grapes
12pm – 175 calories	Simple Cucumber Tomato Salad
2pm – 630 calories	6 medium bananas
5pm – 265 calories	4 dates and ½ cup raisins
7pm – 650 calories	2 medium baked sweet potatoes w/ Cashew Cream

Day 3 – 1775 calories

9am – 270 calories	Date Beverage or other Hot Beverage
12pm – 285 calories	1 pound cherries
2pm – 315 calories	1 pound of grapes
5pm – 550 calories	10 dried smyrna figs
7pm – 355 calories	No Oil No Salt Lentil Soup

Day 4 – 2095 calories

9am – 285 calories	1 pound cherries
12pm – 630 calories	6 medium bananas
2pm – 255 calories	5 peaches
5pm – 550 calories	10 dried smyrna figs
7pm – 375 calories	Maple Pecan Baked Sweet Potato

Day 5 – 1865 calories

9am – 270 calories	Date Beverage or other Hot Beverage
12pm – 315 calories	1 pound of grapes
2pm – 550 calories	10 dried smyrna figs
7pm – 730 calories	Creamy Tomato Soup and Side Salad

Day 6 – 1880 calories

9am – 270 calories	Date Beverage or other Hot Beverage
12pm – 420 calories	4 medium bananas
2pm – 255 calories	5 peaches
5pm – 285 calories	1 pound cherries
7pm – 650 calories	Baked Sweet Potato w/ Cashew Cream

Day 7 – 1760 calories

9am – 255 calories	5 peaches
12pm – 315 calories	1 pound of grapes
2pm – 285 calories	1 pound cherries
5pm – 550 calories	10 dried smyrna figs
7pm – 355 calories	No Oil No Salt Pea Soup

Recipes

Juices

Green Apple Juice
440 calories

4-6 apples
1 cucumber
4 stalks celery
2 cups baby spinach
1 lemon

Simple Green Juice
450 calories

4-6 apples
1 head celery
1-2 lemons

Orange Juice
540 calories

10-12 oranges

Orange Grapefruit
560 calories

2 grapefruits
8 oranges

Orange Lime
510 calories

10 oranges
1 lime

Watermelon Juice
240-320 calories

6 cups of watermelon, juiced or blended

Cucumber Refresher
530 calories

2 cucumbers
6 apples, 3 green, 3 red or your
  favorite variety
1 lemon with peel on

Smoothies

Banana Mylk
630 calories

5-6 bananas
1-2 cups water or water plus ice as desired

Start with 1 cup and add water as desired to get to your preferred thickness. If you prefer a really thick milkshake consistency then start with ½ cup of water or add additional bananas.

Orange Juicius
540 calories

4 bananas
2 oranges
¼ vanilla bean scraped or 1 tsp
 vanilla extract *
1 cup ice
1 cup water

Cherry Smoothie
615 calories

4 bananas
2 cups frozen sweet cherries
1 cup water

Strawberry Banana Smoothie
520 calories

4 bananas
2 cups strawberries (fresh or frozen)
1 cup water or water + ice as desired

Ultimate Refresher
315 calories

1 cup frozen cherries
2 cups fresh grapes
Juice of 1-3 limes

Pumpkin Smoothie
500 calories

4 bananas
¾-1 cup raw pumpkin
½ cup almond milk (or other
 homemade plant milk)(optional –
 not ideal food combining)
1 tsp cinnamon *
1 tsp nutmeg *
5 medjool dates

Breakfast

Just Bananas Pancakes

180 calories per pancake

2 small bananas per pancake

Chop bananas into small pieces. Continue to chop until the banana becomes semi-liquid but there are still small pieces evenly throughout. Place on a dehydrator sheet, shaping into a round about 4 inches wide, and dehydrate at 105 for 8-12 hours, flip and dehydrate 2-3 hours more. The pancakes should be firm on the outside but slightly moist on the inside.

(I usually make them at dinner the night before and dehydrate them overnight, then flip in the morning and enjoy them in the late morning.)

Raw Cinnamon Rolls

150 calories per roll

8 bananas, dehydrated overnight
1 cup dates, soaked 15 minutes
1 tsp cinnamon * (optional)

Slice bananas lengthwise in long strips, 3 strips per banana. Dehydrate for 12 hours.

Soak dates. Drain but reserve liquid. Process dates until smooth adding water 1 tablespoon at a time until smooth and about the consistency of thick jam. Add cinnamon as desired.

Take one banana slice, and spread date mixture about ⅛ inch thick on ¾ of the banana leaving about 1 inch bare at the top. Roll from the date spread end towards the bare end, creating a spiral shape that resembles a cinnamon bun.

Raw Oatmeal

345 calories

2 apples
1 banana
1 tbsp golden flax seed, ground
2 tsp cinnamon *
Water to blend

In a food processor combine all ingredients, starting with 1 tablespoon of water and adding more as needed to blend. Blend until well combined but not completely smooth. Put in a bowl and top with dried fruits if desired. Let sit for 2-3 minutes to thicken.

Pineapple Donut Holes

Makes 4 servings, 370 calories per serving

2 cups dried pineapple
Juice of 1 lime
2 cups dates
1 cup coconut shredded
Extra coconut to roll

Combine all 4 ingredients in food processor and process until well combined and they start to form a ball. For best results start with room temperature dates. If needed add 1-2 tbsp water if the dates are dry. Roll into balls about 1 inch round and then roll in extra coconut to coat.

Raw Bagels with Cream "Cheese"

Makes 8 servings, 390 calories per serving, including Raw Cream Cheese

1½ cups raw cashews

1 cup almonds

1 medium apple, peeled, cored, and sliced

1 tsp ground chia seeds

1 tbsp onion powder (optional) *

¼ cup sesame seeds (optional)

¼ cup poppy seeds (optional)

In a food processor, grind cashews and almonds into a medium-fine powder. Do not over process. If oil is released from the nuts you have gone too far. Add apples, onion powder and chia seeds. Process until the dough ball forms. In a small bowl or plate combine the sesame seeds and poppy seeds. Divide dough into 8 portions and roll into balls. Flatten balls. Using a chopstick, press a hole in the center and go around slowly to widen the hole with the chopstick until it is about as wide as your finger. Press the bagel into the sesame poppy seed mixture on one side. Serve with Raw Cream Cheese or your favorite raw jam.

Raw Cream "Cheese"
1¼ cups cashews

3 tbsp lemon juice

1 tbsp apple cider vinegar *

⅛-¼ cup water as needed

Blend all ingredients until smooth and creamy.

Salads

Simple Salad

170 calories

1 head of iceberg lettuce

3 tomatoes on the vine

Chop finely and add your favorite dressing.

Simple Cucumber Tomato Salad

175 calories

1 head iceberg lettuce

1 medium cucumber

3 medium tomatoes

Chop finely and add your favorite dressing.

Simple Avocado Salad

340 calories

1 avocado, diced

1 medium cucumber, diced

3 medium tomatoes, diced

Dress with juice of 1 or 2 limes

Simple Salad Romaine

530 calories

1 head of romaine lettuce, or 3 romaine hearts
1 cucumber, diced or shredded
1 zucchini, diced or shredded

Dressing
¼ cup cashews
1 red bell pepper
2 dates

Simple Salad with Sweet Red Pepper Dressing

440 calories

1 head lettuce
4 medium tomatoes

Sweet Red Pepper Dressing
1 red bell pepper
4 medjool dates
juice of 1 lemon

Side Salad

165 calories

½ head iceberg lettuce
1 cup frozen peas, warmed on the stove or in warm water

Zucchini Noodle Salad with Sweet Tomato Dressing

335 calories

2 medium zucchini, spiralized or shredded

Sweet Tomato Dressing
3 medium tomatoes
3 dates
1 stalk celery (optional)
juice of 1 lemon (optional)

Spinach Salad

285 calories

1 head romaine lettuce
1 10 oz container baby spinach
1 pound tomatoes
1 medium cucumber, sliced

Dressing optional – Choices include:
    a squeeze of lemon or lime juice
    avocado blended with lemon or lime and ¼ cup water
    3 tomatoes + 3-4 stalks celery blended
    tomato blended with mango
    blueberries or other berries blended with dates.

Classic Salad

400 calories

1 head iceberg lettuce, finely diced
1 head romaine lettuce, finely diced
4-5 tomatoes
3 stalks of celery, diced
1 cucumber, sliced or shredded
1 zucchini, sliced or shredded

This makes a large salad that will feed 1-2 hygienists, 2-4 people transitioning, or 4-6 as a side salad.

Tomato, Cucumber, and Zucchini Salad

190 calories

Chop, shred or spiralize 2 medium zucchini and 1 large cucumber
Dice 4-6 vine ripe tomatoes
juice of 1 lemon, lime, or orange

Kale & Brussels Sprout Salad with Lemon Mustard Dressing

415 calories

5-6 leaves kale, shredded
10 brussels sprouts, shredded
1 apple, shredded
½ head of green cabbage, shredded

Lemon Mustard Dressing

2 tbsp mustard *
2 lemons, zested and squeezed
4-5 medjool dates

Blend all ingredients, add water 1-2 tbsp at a time as needed to blend. (For a non-irritant option simply omit the mustard and add a little extra water.)

Kale Salad with Sweet Orange Dressing

730 calories

1 bunch kale, finely shredded
½ head green cabbage, shredded
¼ cup raisins, mulberries, cherries, or other dried fruit of your choice

Sweet Orange Dressing

4-6 oranges
4 dates

Blend oranges with dates. Combine remaining ingredients in a large bowl. Pour over dressing. Let sit for 5-10 minutes to soften the greens.

Quinoa and Lentil Salad with Sunflower Seed dressing
980 calories

1 head romaine lettuce
1 cup cooked quinoa
1 cup lentils, boiled
2 medium tomatoes
1 red bell pepper

Sunflower Seed Dressing
¼ cup sunflower seeds
juice of 1 large lemon
2 medjool dates
¼ -½ cup water

Salad Dressings and Sauces

These are all assumed to need blending, preferably in a powerful blender like a Vitamix but a normal blender or even food processor will do, will give slightly varying texture.

Basic Cashew Dressing

190 calories

¼ cup cashews
juice of 1 lemon or 1 lime
¼ to ½ cup water depending on preferred texture

Optional:
2-3 dates for a sweeter dressing (less ideal food combining) (adds 60 calories per date)
Fresh or sundried tomatoes
Culinary herbs * (minor irritants): basil, cilantro, dill, garlic powder, onion powder
Classic combinations: sun dried tomatoes + basil *, cilantro * + lime, ranch dressing * (garlic powder, onion powder, fresh parsley, dill, cilantro, lemon juice, black pepper)

Sunflower Seed Dressing

225 calories

¼ cup sunflower seeds
juice of 1-2 lemons
¼ -½ cup water

Blend ¼ cup water, lemon juice and seeds until very smooth. Add additional water to thin to your desired consistency.

Cashew Mayo

Full recipe 1710 calories, 1 tbsp 60 calories

1 ¾ cup raw soaked cashews
¼ cup hemp seeds
3 large dates or 5 small
4 tbsp apple cider vinegar *
juice from 1 whole lemon
pinch of chili powder * (optional)

Avocado Dressing

Full recipe 250 calories

4 Servings 60 calories per serving
1 avocado
juice of 1 lime or lemon
¼ cup water

Optional:
   1 handful of cilantro * (mild irritant)
   1-2 dates for a sweeter dressing
   1 stalk celery for a saltier dressing
   (optional sub 1 zucchini for ½ avocado for a lighter version with less fat)

Simple Salad Dressing

345 calories

¼ cup cashews
1 red bell pepper
2 medjool dates

Blend until smooth.

Orange Cashew Dressing

Full recipe 940 calories
4 servings 235 calories per serving

2 cups of freshly squeezed orange juice
1 cup of cashews (or less)
handful of parsley * (optional)
pinch of dulce * (optional)
Optional: Add celery, sun dried tomatoes, dates, or herbs for different variations.

Savory Tomato Dressing

100 calories

4 tomatoes
2-4 stalks celery

Sweet Tomato Dressing

230 calories

4 tomatoes
2 dates
1 stalk celery

Strawberry Dressing

210 calories

2 medjool dates
1 cup of frozen (thawed) or fresh strawberries
½ cup freshly squeezed lime juice
1 tbsp fresh or dried basil * (optional)

Mango Dressing

400 calories

Blend 2-3 mangos. That's it. Easy peasy.

Tomato Mango Dressing

245 calories

2 tomatoes with 1-2 mangos. Dates optional.

Blueberry Dressing

350 calories

1 cup blueberries
4-5 medjool dates

Red Bell Pepper Vinaigrette

390 calories

2-4 red bell peppers
heavy splash of apple cider vinegar *
4-6 medjool dates

Hygienic Red Bell Pepper Dressing

390 calories

2 red bell peppers
2 large tomatoes
4-6 medjool dates
lemon juice (optional – omit for a sweeter dressing, add for a tangy dressing)

Creamy Tomato Dressing

290 calories

4-5 vine ripe tomatoes
2-4 stalks celery
¼ cup cashews or sunflower seeds
Optional – juice of one lemon
Optional – 2-4 medjool dates (less ideal food combining, but minimal burden;
    adds 65 calories per date)

Hemp Caesar Dressing

Full recipe 840 calories
4 servings 210 calories per serving

½ cup soaked cashews
½ cup hemp seeds
½ cup water
¼ cup apple cider vinegar * (optional)
juice from ½ lemon
½ tsp of coconut or liquid aminos * (optional)
½ tbsp dijon mustard * (optional)

Blend until smooth.

Creamy Cucumber Dressing

260 calories

1 cucumber
¼ cup sunflower seeds
1 lemon, juiced
1 tsp white miso * (optional)

Fat Free Mandarin Twist Dressing

395 calories

5-6 dates
splash apple cider vinegar *
juice of 1 lemon
1 mandarin orange (use regular orange if no mandarin)
½ tsp paprika * (optional)
⅛ tsp chili powder * (optional)

Sunflower Dressing (Transitional)
Full recipe 1120 calories
4 servings 280 calories per serving

1 cup of soaked sunflower seeds
3-4 medjool dates
juice of 1 lemon
half a raw carrot
1 tsp onion powder* (optional)
small handful parsley * (optional)
dash of chili * (optional)
dash of dulse flakes * (optional)
water to desired consistency – appx. ½ cup

Zoodles & Coodles

Zoodles with Marinara
600 calories

2-3 medium zucchini, spiralized

Sauce
5-6 vine ripe tomatoes
4-5 sundried tomatoes
juice of 1 lemon
1 stalk of celery
5-6 medjool dates

Blend all sauce ingredients, and pour over zucchini noodles. Serve immediately.

Sweet Marinara
530 calories

5 vine ripe tomatoes
1-3 stalks of celery
6-10 medjool dates
juice of 1 lemon (or more to your taste)

Start with 1 stalk of celery and 2-3 dates and then add more celery if you prefer a more savory/salty sauce and more dates if you prefer a more sweet sauce. Sun dried tomatoes can be substituted for dates if you prefer no sweetness.

Coodles with Mango Tomato Sauce

545 calories

2-3 cucumbers, spiralized

> *Sauce:*
> 2 tomatoes
> 2 mangoes
>
> Blend tomatoes and mangoes and pour over cucumber noodles. Serve immediately.

Coodles with Avocado Sauce

375 calories

2-3 cucumbers, spiralized

> *Sauce:*
> 1 avocado
> juice of 1 lime
> juice of 1 orange
>
> Blend sauce ingredients and pour over cucumber noodles. Serve immediately.

Raw Soups

Classic Tomato Soup
530 calories

8 tomatoes
5-6 dates
juice of 1 lemon
2 stalks celery

Blend until very smooth. Blend for 1-2 minutes for a warm soup. Top with chopped veggies of your choice, optional.

Creamy Tomato Soup
550 calories

6 tomatoes
¼ cup tahini
5-6 sundried tomatoes
juice of 1 lemon
2 stalks celery
Optional: fresh basil *

Blend all ingredients until very smooth. Blend for 1-2 minutes for a warm soup. Optionally top with fine shredded basil as a garnish.

Spinach Soup
340 calories

1 avocado
4-5 handfuls spinach
juice of 1 lime
½-¾ cup water
1 zucchini
1 cucumber
1 tomato

Blend avocado, spinach, and lime juice with ½ cup water. Add additional water to reach desired thickness keeping in mind that cucumber and zucchini will release water. Finely dice zucchini, cucumber and tomato. Pour avocado mixture in a bowl, and top with diced veggies.

Cucumber Soup
415 calories

¼ cup tahini
juice of 1 large lemon
2-3 stalks celery
1 large cucumber finely diced
3 tsp fresh mint * finely diced

Blend tahini, lemon, and celery until smooth. Place cucumber in a bowl, top with blended mixture, and garnish with fresh mint (optional).

Corn Soup

670 calories

Meat from 1 young thai coconut + ¼ cup water
   OR ¼ cup dehydrated raw coconut shreds + 1 cup water
5-6 ears of corn
1 stalk celery
juice of 1 lime

Remove corn from the cob. Place half of the corn in a serving bowl and another half in the blender. Add to the blender coconut, water, lime juice, and celery. Blend until very smooth. Add to a bowl with the corn. Optional additional toppings: Finely diced cucumber or zucchini, avocado, tomatoes, bell peppers.

Pea Soup

490 calories without toppings

2 cups fresh or frozen peas
1 small avocado or 1 zucchini for a low-fat version
juice of 1 lime
½ cup water

> *Toppings:*
> diced cucumber
> zucchini
> tomatoes
> corn
> pumpkin or sunflower seeds
> or your favorite veggies

Set ½ cup of peas aside, and blend the rest of the peas with water, avocado/zucchini, and lime juice. Pour into a bowl, and top with remaining peas and optional topping vegetables.

Raw Asparagus Soup
260 calories without toppings

¾ cup water
¼ cup sunflower seeds
1 cup chopped asparagus (save the tips for garnish)
1 tsp dry dill
juice of 1 lemon
1 stalk celery
½ small zucchini

Combine all ingredients in the blender and blend until very smooth.

Toppings:
asparagus tips (reserved from above)
fresh corn
diced cucumber
fresh peas (or frozen defrosted)

Top with some or all of the above, diced finely or add your favorite toppings.

Creamy Red Bell Pepper Soup
300 calories

2 red bell peppers
¼ cup sunflower seeds
1 carrot
1 stalk celery
juice of 1 lemon
1 cup warm water

Combine all ingredients in the blender, blend until smooth. Optional: top with diced cucumber, shredded carrot, diced avocado, diced zucchini, sunflower seeds, pumpkin seeds, sesame seeds or your favorite veggies.

Nut Butters and Jams

Peanut Butter

Full recipe 840 calories
1 tbsp 80 calories, ¼ cup 210 calories

1 cup raw spanish peanuts

Place peanuts in the food processor and run for 2-3 minutes. Scrape the bowl and run again for 2-3 minutes. Let the processor cool down. Continue to run in 2-3 minute increments scraping the bowl in between until a smooth butter is formed. It will get dry and crumbly first but will eventually turn into smooth peanut butter. No need to add anything else to it.

Cashew Butter

Full recipe 720 calories
1 tbsp 77 calories, ¼ cup 180 calories

1 cup raw cashews

Place cashews in the food processor and run for 2-3 minutes. Scrape the bowl and run again for 2-3 minutes. Let the processor cool down. Continue to run in 2-3 minute increments scraping the bowl in between until a smooth butter is formed. It will get dry and crumbly first but will eventually turn into smooth cashew butter. No need to add anything else to it.

Sunflower Butter

Full recipe 820 calories
1 tbsp 82 calories, ¼ cup 205 calories

1 cup raw sunflower seeds

Place sunflower seeds in the food processor and run for 2-3 minutes. Scrape the bowl and run again for 2-3 minutes. Let the processor cool down. Continue to run in 2-3 minute increments scraping the bowl in between until a smooth sunflower butter is formed. It will get dry and crumbly first but will eventually turn into smooth sunflower butter. No need to add anything else to it.

Pumpkin Butter Jam

Full recipe 430 calories, 1 tbsp 10 calories

2 cups pie pumpkin
1 apple
½ cup dates
1 tsp pumpkin spice seasoning *
⅓ cup apple juice

Blend until very smooth.

Blueberry Chia Jam

Full recipe 450 calories, 1 tbsp 23 calories

1 cup blueberries
3-4 medjool dates
2 tbsp chia seeds

Blend blueberries with dates, and stir in chia seeds. Let sit for 15 minutes to thicken.

Cheeses

Cashew Cheese

Full recipe 730 calories, 1 tbsp 35 calories

1 cup cashews
juice of 1 lemon
1 tsp apple cider vinegar * (optional)
water as needed to blend

Combine all ingredients in a blender and blend until smooth. Optional, leave at room temperature overnight to ferment creating a more cheese-like flavor.

Red Pepper Cashew Cheese

Full recipe 760 calories, 1 tbsp 37 calories

1 cup cashews, soaked 1 hour (reserve water for blending)
1 red bell pepper
juice of 1 lime

Strain cashews, reserving water. Combine all ingredients plus 2-3 tbsp water, blend until smooth adding water as needed.

Tomato Basil Cheese

Full recipe 770 calories, 1 tbsp 38 calories

1 cup cashews, soaked 1 hour
5 sundried tomatoes
5-6 fresh basil leaves * (or 1 tsp dried) (optional)
juice of 1 lemon

Strain cashews, reserving water. Combine all ingredients plus 2-3 tbsp water, blend until smooth adding water as needed.

Snacks / Appetizers

Apples with Date Caramel
1040 calories

4 apples, sliced in wedges
10 medjool dates or 20 deglet dates, soaked in 1 cup of water for 10-15 minutes
    to soften, reserve water for blending

In a food processor or blender process the soaked dates with ¼ cup of soak water, add additional water 1 tablespoon at a time until you reach your desired consistency.

Zucchini Chips and "Salsa"
20 calories per average zucchini

Thinly slice 3-4 zucchini into rounds and serve with your choice of salsa or other dip recipes below.

Classic Salsa
100 calories
(Transitional – contains some irritants)

2-3 vine ripe tomatoes
1 bell pepper *
1 small sweet onion or shallot *
1 bunch cilantro *
juice of 1-2 limes

Pulse in the food processor until desired texture is reached.

Hygienic Salsa

130 calories

3-5 tomatoes
juice of 1 lime
3-4 stalks of celery
1 red, orange, or yellow bell pepper

Pulse in the food processor until desired texture is reached.

Pumpkin Chia Pudding

400 calories

¼ cup chia seeds
¼ cup coconut water
¼ cup pumpkin purée (blend pumpkin meat with little water and a couple dates
    in blender prior)
¼ cup unsweetened hemp or almond milk (best made at home to avoid
    preservatives)
1 large medjool date (chopped)
coconut flakes for topping
pinch of cardamom * (optional)
½ tsp pumpkin pie spice * or allspice * or cinnamon * (optional)

Blend all ingredients except coconut. Add coconut flakes to top. Let set for 30 minutes or overnight

Mango Pudding
400 to 600 calories

2-3 mangoes of choice

Peel and blend mangoes until smooth. Enjoy!

Stuffed Mini Sweet Peppers
Full recipe 1080 calories
4 servings 270 calories per serving

1 bag mini bell peppers
1 cup sunflower seeds, soaked 15 minutes to soften
1 red or orange bell pepper
2-3 sundried tomatoes, soaked for 15 minutes
juice of 1 lemon or lime

Strain sunflower seeds and sundried tomatoes but retain water from sundried tomatoes. Combine all ingredients in a food processor. Process until fairly smooth or chunky, as you prefer. Add tomato soak water as needed to reach desired consistency. Slice peppers in half and remove seeds and stem. Lay on a serving platter and fill with sunflower spread.

Raw Stuffed Mushrooms

Full recipe 860 calories

If 2 servings 430 calories each, if 4 servings 215 calories each

1 box cremini mushrooms

2 tbsp Bragg Liquid Aminos *

Cashew Cream

1 cup cashews

juice of 2 small lemons

½ cup water or more to desired consistency

Pesto

2 cups baby spinach or baby kale

½ cup sunflower seeds

4-6 large basil leaves *

1 tsp lemon zest

juice of ½ a lemon

Clean mushrooms, remove the stems and discard or save for raw veggie burgers, place mushroom tops in a small container with Bragg Liquid Aminos, place lid on container and shake well to coat the mushrooms. Set aside to marinate, shaking the container every few minutes to distribute the Braggs.

Cashew Cream: In a food processor or blender, combine the cashews, lemon juice and water and process until very smooth. Set aside.

Pesto: In the food processor combine the baby spinach and/or baby kale, sunflower seeds, basil, lemon zest and lemon juice. Process until well combined but with a little texture.

Assembly: Lay out mushrooms upside down on a serving tray. Taking a small spoon, scoop the pesto into the cavity in the mushroom. Evenly distribute pesto across all mushrooms. Then top with a dollop of cashew cream. Serve at room temperature, or dehydrate for 2-3 hours to warm.

Dips and Spreads

Simple Holiday Dip
135 calories

2 tbsp of hemp seeds
1 cup peel zucchini

Blend hemp seeds and zucchini. Cut carrot, cucumber, bell pepper and celery to dip into this creamy sauce.

Asparagus Dip
Full recipe 870 calories, 1 tbsp 25 calories

1 bunch asparagus, rough chopped, save the tips for mixing in at the end
½ cup sunflower seed butter
juice 1-2 lemons, to taste

In a food processor add asparagus, saving the tops to add later, add sunflower butter and juice of 1 lemon. Process until smooth and creamy. Taste and add more lemon as needed to reach desired taste. Add water as needed to thin to desired consistency. Serve with sliced cucumbers, zucchini, bell peppers, celery, or raw crackers.

Green Pea Dip
Full recipe 500 calories

2 servings 250 calories per serving
1 cup green peas, fresh or frozen
½ cup raw almonds
juice of 1 lime
⅓ cup fresh cilantro * (optional)

Place almonds in a food processor and process until medium fine. Add remaining ingredients and process until smooth.

Sunflower Pâté

Full recipe 880 calories

4 servings 220 calories per serving
1 cup sunflower seeds, soaked 15 minutes to soften
1 red or orange bell pepper
2-3 sundried tomatoes, soaked for 15 minutes
juice of 1 lemon or lime

Strain sunflower seeds and sundried tomatoes but retain water from sundried tomatoes. Combine all ingredients in a food processor. Process until roughly chopped for use in sushi rolls or raw sandwiches/wraps. Process until smooth for a dip or salad dressing. Add tomato soak water as needed to reach desired consistency.

Hummus

480 calories

1 cup dried sprouted chickpeas
⅛ cup tahini
juice of 1-2 lemons
paprika * and oil * (optional)

Soak 1 cup dried sprouted chickpeas for several hours or overnight. Normal chickpeas can be used, but they should be cooked* first (boil for 20-30 minutes) to help reduce starchiness. Can also use boiling water to soak in order to reduce soak time. Set water aside and place chickpeas into a high-speed blender with tahini. Add lemon juice as the mixture becomes unable to blend. You may need to add a small quantity of water – try to blend as much as you can and then add water as the mixture becomes too thick to blend any further. If you're using oil then you can add some oil as the hummus is blending then a little more on top as a finisher.

Butternut Squash Hummus
420 calories

1 cup of soaked / sprouted chickpeas (soak for a couple days in advance)
1 cup of butternut squash purée
1 tbsp of tahini
½ tsp cumin * (optional)

Blend on high speed in powerful blender until warmed and smooth.

Happy Pâté
420 calories

1 red bell pepper
2 small carrots
1 tomato
¼ cup almonds soaked for 2 hours
2 medjool dates, pitted
juice of 1 lemon

Combine all ingredients in a food processor or blender and process until smooth. Add water as needed to blend 1 tablespoon at a time.

Pesto (oil-free)
440 calories

3 cups basil *
¼ cup sunflower seeds
¼ cup walnuts
1 stalk celery
1-2 large kale leaves *
¾ cup water

Process until desired texture is reached.

Side Dishes

Cauliflower Mash w/ Mushroom Gravy

Full recipe 1350 calories

4 servings 340 calories per serving

1 head cauliflower

½ cup pine nuts

1 cup cashews

2 tbsp white miso *

1 tsp garlic powder *

2 tbsp lemon juice or water

In a food processor combine all ingredients and process until smooth.

Mushroom Gravy

1 8 oz container cremini mushrooms

2 tbsp Bragg Liquid Aminos *

1 tsp rubbed sage *

½ tsp thyme *

½ tsp rosemary *

¼-½ cup water

Combine ¼ cup water with remaining ingredients and blend until very smooth, thin to desired consistency with remaining water.

Raw Stuffing

650 calories

1 cup mushrooms
2 tbsp Bragg Liquid Aminos *
2 stalks celery
2 small carrots
½ cup pecans
2 dates
1 small head of cauliflower
½ tsp rosemary *
½ tsp sage *
½ tsp thyme *
¼ tsp nutmeg *

Marinate mushrooms in Bragg Liquid Aminos, set aside. In the food processor, process cauliflower until it is roughly the size of rice grains. Place in a medium sized bowl and set aside. Process pecans, dates, marinated mushrooms and spices until they form a thick paste. Stir together mushroom mixture with cauliflower until well combined. Process carrots until finely chopped. Hand chop celery into small pieces. Stir in carrots and celery. Serve at room temperature, or warm slightly in the dehydrator.

Raw Cranberry Sauce

680 calories

16 oz bag fresh cranberries
zest of 1 orange
½ cup orange juice (or more as desired for a thinner sauce)
1 cup dates – soaked in warm water for 10 minutes

Drain dates, combine all ingredients in a food processor, and process until chunky.

Entrees

Fajitas

350 calories

1 red bell pepper
1 orange bell pepper
1 yellow bell pepper
1 portobello mushroom
1 ear of fresh sweet corn
1 head of romaine lettuce
juice of 1 lime
Optional: chili powder *, taco seasoning (salt-free version) *, cilantro *,
    avocado, liquid smoke *

Thinly slice the mushroom and squeeze the lime juice over top. Let sit while you prepare the other ingredients. Thinly slice the bell peppers into strips. Mix with the mushrooms and lime juice. If desired add chili powder or other taco seasonings. Serve with raw salsa, finely diced cilantro, and/or slices of avocado.

Raw Tacos

500 to 1500 calories

1 head romaine lettuce
1 batch hygienic taco filling (see recipe below)
1 batch classic or hygienic salsa (see recipes under Snacks)
1 ear corn

Take a lettuce leaf and top with taco filling, salsa, and corn.

Hygienic Taco Filling

350 calories

1 cup sundried tomatoes, soaked
½ cup dates, soaked
1 tsp paprika *
juice of 1 lime

Classic Taco Filling
1320 calories
1 cup mushrooms
1 cup walnuts
½ pumpkin or sunflower seeds
1 tsp chili powder *
1 tsp onion powder *
1 tsp garlic powder *
1 tbsp Bragg Liquid Aminos *

Taco "Meat"
930 calories

1 cup walnuts
1/2 cup dried mulberries
1/2 cup dried tomatoes
1 cup carrot

Process all ingredients together in a food processor until finely ground but with some texture.

Banana Tacos
Makes 10 tacos, 55 calories each

1 head of romaine
5 bananas

Take a lettuce leaf and top with ½ banana

Optional: Add date sauce, dates or other fruits like berries, mango or pineapple, or substitute other fruits for the bananas.

Mixed Berry Tacos
Makes 10 tacos, 75 calories each

1 head romaine lettuce
2 cups mixed berries
5 bananas

Take a lettuce leaf and top with ½ banana, add mixed berries.

Collard Wraps
300-500 calories

1-2 large collard leaves per person
2 tbsp sunflower pâté
shredded lettuce
Your choice of 2-3 vegetables, shredded or chopped, including avocado, zucchini, cucumbers, bell peppers, tomatoes, carrots, cabbage, brussels sprouts, alfalfa sprouts, broccoli sprouts, asparagus, etc.

Take a collard leaf and lay it on the cutting board. Remove the stem of the leaf by holding your knife parallel to the cutting board and cutting away most of the thick central vein of the leaf so it rolls more easily. With the light underside of the leaf facing up, spread some sunflower pâté on the bottom ⅓ of the leaf. Add the remaining toppings on top of the pâté, keeping everything on the bottom ⅓. Fold in the sides then roll like a burrito keeping the sides tucked in as you roll.

Raw Plant-Based Sushi Rolls
320 calories

Option 1

2 sheets of nori * (untoasted preferably)
1 cucumber, sliced into matchsticks
1 zucchini, sliced into matchsticks
1 avocado, sliced into matchsticks
2 romaine leaves or 2 small handfuls of mixed baby greens or spinach

Lay the nori sheet on a cutting board. Lay lettuce across the nori. Add remaining toppings onto the lettuce. Lightly wet the top strip of nori that is not covered with toppings. Roll tightly pressing the seal at the top. Set the seal side down for 2-3 minutes before slicing. Using a very sharp knife, slice into 6 slices about 1 inch thick.

Option 2

Sunflower Pâté (see recipe under Dips and Spreads)
2 romaine leaves or 2 small handfuls of mixed baby greens or spinach
1 cucumber, sliced into matchsticks
1 zucchini, sliced into matchsticks

Lay the nori sheet on a cutting board. Spread sunflower pâté across nori leaving the top 1-1.5 inches bare. Lay lettuce across the pâté on the bottom ⅓. Add remaining toppings onto the lettuce. Lightly wet the top strip of nori that is not covered with toppings. Roll tightly pressing the seal at the top. Set the seal side down for 2-3 minutes before slicing. Using a very sharp knife, slice into 6 slices about 1 inch thick.

Option 3

dates (soaked 15 minutes), sliced into matchsticks
red bell pepper, sliced into matchsticks
cucumber, sliced into matchsticks
sundried tomato (soaked 15 minutes), sliced into matchsticks

Lay the nori sheet on a cutting board. Arrange toppings across the bottom 1/3rd. Lightly wet the top strip of nori that is not covered with toppings. Roll tightly pressing the seal at the top. Set the seal side down for 2-3 minutes before slicing. Using a very sharp knife, slice into 6 slices about 1 inch thick.

Option 4

½ head cauliflower
2 tbsp ground flax seeds
1 cucumber, sliced into matchsticks
1 zucchini, sliced into matchsticks
1 avocado, sliced into matchsticks

In a food processor combine cauliflower and flax seeds, and process until cauliflower reaches the consistency of rice. Lay the nori sheet on a cutting board. Spread cauliflower on the sheet leaving about 1 inch to 1.5 inches at the top clear. Add remaining toppings to the bottom ⅓. Lightly wet the top strip of nori that is not covered with toppings. Roll tightly pressing the seal at the top. Set the seal side down for 2-3 minutes before slicing. Using a very sharp knife, slice into 6 slices about 1 inch thick.

Veggie Burgers

Full recipe 1100 calories
4 Servings 275 calories per serving

1 cup pecans
1 carrot
1 stalk celery
4-5 sundried tomatoes, soaked 15 minutes
2 medjool dates
2 tbsp flax seeds, ground
1 tomato
1 red or orange bell pepper

Combine all ingredients in a food processor and process until fine dice and mixture comes together. Form into patties about 3 inches wide and ½ thick. Serve immediately or dehydrate for 4-5 hours, flipping once for a crispy outside.

Serve alone or on lettuce leaves, bell pepper slices or portobello mushrooms as bread.

Veggie Sandwiches

400-600 calories

red bell peppers, 1 per sandwich
1-2 leaves of lettuce per sandwich
1 cucumber, sliced
1 vine ripe tomato, sliced
Your choice of dip, pâté, cashew "cheese" or spread

Slice the sides off of each bell pepper to make large slabs. These will be your bread. Spread with your choice of dip, pâté, cashew "cheese", or spread on one half of the bell pepper. Top with tomatoes, lettuce, and cucumber. Add the second half as the top slice of bread.

Zucchini Ravioli with Marinara Sauce

Full recipe 1900 calories, 3 servings 633 calories per serving

The ravioli is prepared by using a vegetable peeler and peeling long strips of zucchini. To make a ravioli, criss-cross 2 strips with two strips making a "T". Add a spoonful of filling and fold all four sides in to make a square little ravioli – repeat until all filling is used. I peel approximately 3 medium sized zucchinis (20 calories per average zucchini).

Ravioli Filling (1610 calories)

1 ¼ cup soaked raw cashews (soak1 hour)

3/4 cup hemp seeds

1/4 cup lemon juice

1/4 cup water

1 tbsp of miso (optional, not hygienic)

Once you've filled a small square baking dish with ravioli, add the raw marinara sauce (this sauce can be used on top of plain zucchini noodles as well).

Raw Marinara Sauce (230 calories)

1 pound tomatoes (roma, grape or cherry, on the vine, etc.), chopped

1 cup (3 oz) sun-dried tomatoes (not in oil)

1 teaspoon garlic powder (optional, not hygienic)

2 tbsp shallots * (optional)

1/2 cup herbs * (cilantro, parsley or basil), medium packed (optional)

Soak sun dried tomatoes an hour prior and drain before using. Blend ingredients together until sauce-like consistency. Serve on top of zucchini noodles also!

Option – Hygienic Raw Sauce (480 calories)

5-6 vine ripe tomatoes

4-5 sundried tomatoes

juice of 1 lemon

1 stalk of celery

5-6 medjool dates

Blend all ingredients until smooth.

Raw Holiday Loaf
1900 calories

Make in advance – Uses Dehydrator

Marinate First:
2 cups portobello or cremini mushrooms, roughly chopped
2 tbsp Bragg Liquid Aminos *

Grind together first:
1 cup almonds
1 cup walnuts
¾ tsp dried thyme *
¼ tsp dried sage *
½ tsp onion powder *
½ tsp garlic powder *
¼ cup chopped parsley *

2 stalks celery, roughly chopped
¼ cup sundried tomatoes, soaked
4 dates, soaked
½ red bell pepper
1 tsp lemon juice

For the best flavor, marinate the mushrooms overnight in the Bragg Liquid Aminos. Grind the nuts and spices in a food processor until fine. Transfer to a bowl and set aside.

Place remaining ingredients in the food processor, including the mushrooms and process until it starts to stick together but there are still some medium fine chunks.

Pour into a bowl with the dry ingredients and knead until well combined. Shape into a rectangular loaf and place in the dehydrator for 8-12 hours.

Dehydrator Recipes

Date Bread Raw

2150 calories

Note: This recipe is versatile and can be made with many other ingredients that you may find suitable.

1 cup of ground flax seeds
1 tbsp olive oil * (optional)
dried or fresh rosemary to taste * (optional)
1 cup of soaked dates
½ cup ground sunflower seeds

Blend all ingredients together in a food processor, Thermomix, or blender, when reaching desired consistency, (usually thick), spread on parchment paper or on dehydrator trays. Dehydrate for 12 hours. Makes a nice flat bread to eat with salads, or to top with lettuce, tomato and avocado!

Raw Wraps

1300 calories

1 cup grated carrot
1 cup grated zucchini, (soak moisture out with a towel)
1 cup of flax meal
2 cups water (use extra if needed)
1 tsp cumin * (optional)
1 tsp smoked paprika * (optional)
1-2 tbsp tamari *(optional)

Place all ingredients into your Vitamix container and secure the lid. Turn your variable speed to 1 and then quickly turn up to speed 10 and then override to HIGH speed. Blend until you get a smooth pancake batter consistency. The consistency will depend on how dry you got your grated carrot and zucchini with the towel. Pour your mixture onto drying sheets that are lining your plastic mesh trays in the dehydrator. Dehydrate 12 hours.
Fill with your favorite toppings, I like to wrap lettuce with tomato and avocado!

Zucchini Chips

350 calories

5-10 zucchini or yellow squash

Optional seasonings * (non-hygienic): chili powder, cayenne, onion powder,
   garlic powder, cumin, black pepper, Bragg Liquid Aminos or tamari

Optional seasonings (hygienic): sesame seeds, poppy seeds, sauce made from
   tomatoes & mango, tomatoes & dates or tomatoes & celery, date syrup
   (dates blended with enough water to thin to desired consistency)

Slice zucchini into ¼-½ inch thick rounds or slice lengthwise into slabs of the same
thickness. Apply sauce or spices as desired. Dehydrate 12-24 hours until crispy.

Corn Chips

1330 calories

2 cups fresh or frozen corn
1 yellow bell pepper
1 cup flax seeds
juice of 1 or 2 limes
1 tsp white miso * (optional)
1-2 medjool dates

Place all ingredients in a blender and blend until smooth. On silicone dehydrator
sheets, form into rounds about 2 inches in diameter and ¼ inch thick. Dehydrate
for 12 hours, flip and dry for 4-5 hours more or until crispy.

Cooked Foods

Vegetable Stock
425 calories

½ head of cabbage
1 pound carrots
1 head celery
rosemary *, thyme * onion powder *, garlic powder *, or your favorite
    herbs/spices * (optional)
mushrooms, fresh or dried (optional)

Combine all ingredients in your largest stock pot and fill with water 1-2 inches below the rim. Let simmer for 1-2 hours. Strain and allow to cool, then store in the fridge for use the same week or in the freezer for later use.

Tomato Vegetable Soup
Full recipe 500 calories
4 servings 125 calories per serving

6-8 roma tomatoes, blended
4 cups Vegetable Stock
½ head cabbage, cut into 1 inch pieces
1 handful green beans, cut into 1 inch pieces or 1 cup peas
1-2 medium carrots, sliced
4 stalks celery, sliced
½ head cauliflower, cut into 1-2 inch pieces
1 bunch kale, swiss chard or collards, shredded or torn into chunks
Optional: fresh basil *, oregano *, thyme *

Combine tomatoes and stock. Bring to a boil and simmer on medium heat while cutting the other vegetables. Add carrots and celery, and simmer for 5 min before adding the remaining vegetables. Cook until the cauliflower is just fork tender.

Roasted Butternut Squash Soup

680 calories

1 large butternut squash * or other winter squash*
1 tbsp olive or coconut oil *
1 pound carrots
2 tbsp fresh or dried sage *
4 cups low sodium or no salt added vegetable broth * (store-bought or make
    your own from recipe)
2 stalks celery

Coat butternut squash lightly with oil and bake at 350 for 20-25 minutes. Remove peel and dice, and set aside. Dice celery, and carrot into a large pot add sage and broth and cook for 20-30 minutes. Add butternut squash. Serve as is or blend for a smooth creamy soup, or blend half and leave half chunky as desired.

Lentil Soup

Full recipe 650 calories
4 servings 160 calories per serving

1 16 oz bag of green/brown lentils *
3-4 large carrots
4 stalks celery
2 tbsp cumin *
4 cups Vegetable Stock *

In a soup pot on medium heat place 3-4 tbsp of vegetable stock. Sauté celery and carrots until lightly brown. Add remaining ingredients, bring to boil, and cook for 25-30 minutes until lentils are tender.

Split Pea Soup

720 calories

1 bag of dried split peas

3-4 large carrots

4 stalks celery

2 tbsp cumin *

4 cups Vegetable Stock *

In a soup pot on medium heat place 3-4 tbsp of vegetable stock Add celery and carrots and cook for 4-5 minutes until lightly brown. Add remaining ingredients, bring to boil, and cook for 25-30 minutes until peas are tender.

Black Bean Soup

Full recipe 940 calories

4 servings 235 calories per serving

1 16 oz bag black beans *, soaked overnight

3-4 roma tomatoes

2 red bell peppers

3-4 large carrots

4 stalks celery

2 tbsp chili powder *

1 tsp cayenne * (optional)

1 tbsp cumin *

4 cups Vegetable Stock *

In a soup pot on medium heat place 3-4 tbsp of vegetable stock. Add celery and carrots and cook for 4-5 minutes until lightly brown. Add remaining ingredients, bring to boil, and cook for 35-45 minutes until beans are tender.

No Oil "Fries"
120 to 160 calories per potato

sweet potatoes, red potatoes, or yukon potatoes*

Optional *: season with rosemary & thyme, taco seasonings, chili powder or your favorite spices/herbs (*)

Preheat the oven to 425. Cut desired serving of potatoes into thin fries or wedges. Place on a baking tray lined with parchment paper or on a silicon baking mat. Bake for 25-30 minutes for thin fries and 30-40 minutes for thicker wedges. Flip halfway through.

Red Lentil Flatbreads
Full recipe 680 calories,
Half recipe 340 calories

1 cup dried red lentils *
2 cups water

Either soak red lentils for several hours or boil water and pour over lentils and soak for 30 minutes. Place lentils and water into a blender and blend until fully broken down into a batter. Fry batter on a nonstick surface over medium heat and flip after 3-5 minutes.

No Salt, No Oil Vegetable Stock

For Soups And Flavoring Quinoa, Bean Or Vegetable Dishes
450 calories

Stock can be portioned and frozen for ease of use

1 head of cabbage – green, red, or napa
5-6 carrots
1 head celery
1 8 oz container of mushrooms or package of dried mushrooms – any variety or
   mix more than one kind
2-3 tomatoes

Roughly chop all ingredients and place In your largest stock pot. Fill to 2 inches below the top with water. Boil for 45 minutes to 1 hour. Strain vegetables, leaving stock in pot. (Cooked vegetables can be eaten with a little Bragg Liquid Aminos or add a nut/seed based salad dressing.)

No Oil No Salt Lentil Soup

Makes 6 servings, 355 calories per serving

1 16 oz bag of lentils
4 cups vegetable broth
4 cups water
5 carrots, chopped
5 stalks celery, chopped
3 tomatoes, chopped
2 medium sized potatoes, chopped
2 tbsp of Bragg Liquid Aminos, or more to taste
1-2 tbsp cumin *, to taste

In a large pot, combine all ingredients, bring to a boil and simmer for 45 minutes to one hour.

Creamy Tomato Soup II (Raw or Cooked)

Makes 2 servings, 565 calories per serving

2 pounds tomatoes, roma makes a thicker soup but any variety is fine
1 cup Vegetable Stock or water
2-3 carrots, diced
2-3 stalks celery, diced
Cashew Cream, see below
2 dates
Fresh or dried Italian herbs to taste – basil *, oregano *, thyme * (optional)

Cashew Cream

½ cup of cashews
juice of 1 small lemon
¼ cup water or more to desired consistency

Blend cashew cream ingredients until smooth and creamy then add remaining soup ingredients and blend until smooth. If you prefer a chunkier soup you can leave some of the tomatoes diced and blend half the tomatoes.

This recipe can be served raw, or heated on the stove until warm.

No Oil No Salt Pea Soup

Makes 6 Servings, 355 calories per serving

1 16 oz bag of dried green peas or frozen peas

4 cups vegetable broth

4 cups water

5 carrots, chopped

5 stalks celery, chopped

2 medium sized potatoes, chopped

2 tbsp of Bragg Liquid Aminos, or more to taste

1-2 tbsp smoked paprika * (sweet paprika, not hot)

½ tsp dried thyme * (optional)

½ tsp dried marjoram * (optional)

Or substitute your favorite culinary herbs as desired.

In a large pot, combine all ingredients, bring to a boil and simmer for 45 minutes to one hour.

Hummus

Add to any salad as a calorie boost or pair with soup meals
Full recipe 600 calories
Half recipe 300 calories

2 cups cooked chickpeas *, rinsed and drained

juice of 1 lemon

2 tablespoons tahini

1 tbsp Bragg Liquid Aminos, or to taste as desired

¼ – ½ cup water to desired consistency

Add all ingredients (except water) in order listed to a food processor and begin processing. Add water slowly through the feed tube and process until creamy and desired thickness. Add more water as needed to achieve your desired consistency.

Optional, add sundried tomatoes or your favorite herbs as desired.

Maple Pecan Baked Sweet Potato

375 calories

1 medium sweet potato – appx. 2" by 5"
1 tbsp maple syrup *
¼ cup chopped pecans

Bake sweet potato until tender, top with maple syrup and chopped pecans.

Baked Sweet Potato w/ Cashew Cream

650 calories

2 medium sweet potatoes, baked

Cashew Cream
½ cup of cashews
juice of 1 small lemon
¼ cup water, or more to desired consistency

Blend until smooth.

Top baked sweet potato with Cashew Cream.

Simple Salad with Quinoa and Creamy Tomato Dressing

345 calories

1 head of iceberg lettuce
3 tomatoes on the vine
1 cup cooked quinoa

Creamy Tomato Dressing
¼ cup cashews
juice of 1 lemon or 1 lime
4-6 sundried tomatoes
2 medjool dates
¼ to ½ cup water depending on your preferred texture

Raw Desserts

Banana Nice Cream

400 calories

Slice ripe bananas into small chunks and freeze. Take 2 cups of frozen bananas and place them in the food processor and process until creamy. Eat immediately or keep in the freezer until ready to serve. Best if served within 3 hours.

Optional flavor additions:

carob powder – 2-3 tbsp

½ cup frozen peaches

½ cup frozen cherries

any other frozen fruits of your choice

fresh mint *

cacao nibs * or cacao powder *

maple syrup *

swirl in or top with Date Caramel (see recipe in Raw Desserts)

Mulberry Apple Tarts

Full recipe 2050 calories; 30 tarts 68 calories each

Crust:

2 cups dates

2 cups dried mulberries

1 ½ cups shredded coconut

1 cup coconut flour

Topping:

¼ cup mulberries

Filling:

1 gala apple

1 granny smith apple

1 fuji apple

2 honeycrisp apples

1 cup raisins

1 cup dates

juice of 1 lemon

2 tsp apple pie spice

Crust: Process all 4 ingredients in a food processor until they start to stick together. Press into mini cupcake pans (makes 30 small tarts) or 8" or 9" pie pan for a full-sized pie. Stick in the freezer to set while preparing other ingredients.

Filling: Set aside 1 Honeycrisp apple and raisins. Combine the remaining filling ingredients in the food processor and process until you reach a chunky applesauce consistency. Take the remaining apple and finely chop it to roughly the same size as the raisins. Stir in raisins and chopped apples.

Fill crusts with filling and top with additional mulberries.

Blueberry Pie

Full recipe 2390 calories
If 12 Slices 200 calories each, if 8 Slices 300 calories each

Crust:

1 cup pecans
1 cup almonds
½ cup dates

Filling:

½ cup dates
2 bananas
3 cups blueberries (fresh or frozen)

Crust: Combine pecans and almonds in a food processor and chop for about 30 seconds. Add dates and process until it starts to stick together and form a ball. Pour into the pie pan and press together to form the crust.

Filling: Combine 1 cup of blueberries with the dates and bananas in a blender or food processor, and blend until smooth.

Place the remaining 2 cups of blueberries in the pie pan. Pour the banana mixture over the blueberries. Chill in the fridge for 30 minutes to a few hours before serving. To store, freeze whole pie or individual slices.

Cherry Pie

Full recipe 2400 calories
If 12 Slices 200 calories each, if 8 Slices 300 calories each

Crust:

1 cup pecans
1 cup almonds
½ cup dates

Filling:

½ cup dates
2 bananas
3 cups cherries (fresh or frozen)

Crust: Combine pecans and almonds in a food processor and chop for about 30 seconds. Add dates and process until it starts to stick together and form a ball. Pour into the pie pan and press together to form the crust.

Filling: Combine 1 cup of cherries with the dates and bananas in a blender or food processor and blend until smooth.

Place the remaining 2 cups of cherries in the pie pan. Pour the banana mixture over the cherries. Chill in the fridge for 30 minutes to a few hours before serving. To store, freeze whole pie or individual slices.

Raw Fudge Brownies

Full recipe 1420 calories
If 4 Servings 355 calories each, if 8 Servings 175 calories each

1 cup walnuts
1 cup dates
¼ raw cacao powder * (not hygienic – stimulant) OR ¼ cup raw carob powder (hygienic)

In a food processor, pulse walnuts until fine, about 30 seconds. Do not overprocess as this will release the oils. Add cacao/carob and pulse until combined. Add dates and process until the dough ball forms. Form into a square about ½ inch thick. Slice into squares. Chill for 15-30 minutes before serving or serve at room temperature.

Caramel Pecan Brownies

1835 calories
If 4 Servings 460 calories each, if 8 Servings 230 calories each

Brownie Ingredients:

1 cup walnuts

1 cup dates

½ cup raw cacao powder * OR ½ cup carob powder

Date Caramel: see full recipe below

1 cup dates + water to soak

2-4 tbsp of reserved soak water

Topping:

½ cup pecans

In a food processor, pulse walnuts until fine, about 30 seconds. Do not overprocess as this will release the oils. Add cacao/carob and pulse until combined. Add dates and process until the dough ball forms. Form into a square about ½ inch thick. Top with caramel and pecans. Slice into squares. Chill for 15-30 minutes before serving or serve at room temperature.

Date Caramel

420 calories

1 cup medjool (appx. 6-7) or other dates, soaked 15 minutes, reserve soak water

Blend dates with 2 tbsp water, add more water 1 tablespoon at a time until it reaches the desired consistency, thicker for a dip, thinner for a syrup.

Raw Vegan Brownies

Full recipe 4150 calories

If 10 Servings 415 calories each, if 20 Servings 210 calories each

20 medjool dates

2½ cups almond flour

¼ cup maple syrup * (or homemade date syrup)

½ cup japanese sweet potato * (peeled, chopped and blended first) – OR substitute banana for potato

1 tbsp vanilla extract *

1 cup crushed macadamia nuts

½ cup carob powder

Line a brownie pan with parchment paper. Blend all the ingredients, except for the macadamia nuts, in your food processor until a brownie like batter is formed. Transfer to a mixing bowl and stir in the crushed macadamia nuts. Pour batter into a lined pan and top with extra macadamia nuts. Put into the refrigerator until hardened.

Raw Vegan Carrot Cake with Frosting (optional)

Full recipe 3200 calories

If 12 Servings 260 calories each, if 8 Servings 400 calories each

Carrot Cake (can be made into energy balls if no frosting is desired)

2 cups shredded carrot

2 cups of chopped / pitted medjool dates

2½ cups chopped walnuts (optional)

1 tsp vanilla (optional)

1-2 tsp cinnamon * (optional)

pinch of nutmeg * (optional)

½ cup of shredded coconut

¼ cup raisins

Stir together in a large bowl. Blend the dates in a little bit of water first until smooth / chunky, then add the rest of the ingredients and stir together. Press all ingredients into a baking dish until compacted together. Top with raw cashew icing if desired or eat as is.

Raw Cashew Frosting
1¼ cup soaked raw cashews (drain)
½ cup water
2 tbsp of lemon juice
3 tbsp of maple syrup * (or homemade date syrup)
1 tsp vanilla extract * (optional)

Blend at high speed until creamy and thick. Spread on top of cake, refrigerate until hard and cut into squares and serve.

Raw Pumpkin Pie

Full recipe 2160 calories
If 12 Servings 180 calories each, if 8 Servings 270 calories each

Crust:
Combine equal parts:
1 cup almond flour
1 cup raw applesauce (purée a few dates with apples and a little lemon)

Mix together to form a crust – press into pie pan – let set in the refrigerator for at least an hour before filling.

Filling:
1¾ cup of raw pumpkin purée
¾ cup plant milk
4 dates
1 cup sweetener (date syrup, maple syrup *, etc.)
½ tsp cinnamon * (optional)
2 tsp allspice * (optional. I usually omit cinnamon if using allspice)
1 tsp vanilla extract * (optional)
¼ cup psyllium husk *

Blend everything together until smooth. Pour into pie crust and refrigerate until time to serve. Note: You can fill this crust with any raw, fruity filling such as apples tossed in date syrup & cinnamon (optional, not hygienic).

Lemon Cookies with Blueberry Jam

Full recipe 5040 calories, 20 Cookies 250 calories each

Cookie:

juice of 4 lemons

3 cups shredded coconut

2 cups coconut flour

3 cups dates

Using food processor combine all and process until it forms a dough ball and all dates are well incorporated. Roll into 1 inch balls, press with thumb in center, while building up the sides to form a small cavity.

Jam:

2 pints blueberries

9-10 dates

Blend until smooth, refrigerate until thickens. Spoon filling or use a squeeze bottle to fill the cavities with jam. Top with a blueberry in each cookie.

Raw Cheesecake with Jam or Date Caramel

Full recipe 5600 calories

If 12 Servings 470 calories each, if 8 Servings 700 calories each

Crust:

1 cup pecans

1 cup dates

½ cup shredded raw coconut

Filling:

4 cups cashews, soaked 1-4 hours

⅓ cup coconut oil *

¾ cup lemon juice

¾ cup maple syrup *

1 tbsp vanilla extract *

water as needed to blend – about ¼ to ½ cup

Pick your topping:

Cranberry Topping

1 cup fresh cranberries
4 medjool dates, soaked 10-15 minutes
2-3 tbsp water

Blueberry Topping

1 cup blueberries
3 medjool dates

Date Caramel

20 medjool dates
¼ -½ cup water

Crust: In a food processor combine all three ingredients and process on high until a ball begins to form. For a large cheesecake use a 9 inch springform pan. Press the crust into the pan and use a glass to press until it is even and sticking together well. If your mixture is too dry to stick together on its own add 1-2 additional dates or 1 tablespoon of water while the food processor is running.

For mini cheesecakes you will need a mini cheesecake pan or you could use a mini cupcake pan with cupcake liners and remove the liners before serving. This recipe makes about 30 mini cheesecakes. For the mini pans take about 1 tablespoon of crust mixture and press into the bottom of each hole.

Filling: Combine all ingredients in a blender or a food processor and blend until very smooth, adding water as needed to get it to a smooth creamy texture. You want to add as little water as possible so just add a little at a time.

Topping: Blend all ingredients until smooth. It should be a thick jam. If it is too thin add another date. If it is too thick to blend smoothly add a little more water.

Pour filling over the crust. Then using a spoon scoop about 1 tablespoon of jam on top of each mini cheesecake. If you are making a large cheesecake, place the cheesecake in the freezer for 1 hour before adding the jam so the cheesecake is firm and you can spread the jam. Freeze the cheesecakes for a few hours or until 1 hour before you are ready to serve. Keep in the fridge until you are ready to serve.

Hot Beverages – Coffee and Tea Alternatives

Date Beverage / Date Tea (1 Serving)
270 calories

4 medjool dates or 6-8 smaller dates
8 oz hot water

Remove pits and caps from dates and place in blender with hot water. Blend until smooth and creamy.

Try different flavors: add 1 tablespoon lemon juice, lime juice or orange juice; add banana, apple, mulberries or raisins. Use a little more water when adding dried fruits.

Mock Mocha (1 serving)
280 calories

4 medjool dates or 6-8 smaller dates
1 tbsp raw carob powder
8 oz hot water

Remove pits and caps from dates and place in blender with carob powder and hot water. Blend until smooth and creamy.

If you are not fully ready to stop caffeine, you can use raw cacao powder instead of carob, to step down gradually and avoid headaches.

Coffee Substitute (1 serving)
60 calories

1 tbsp mesquite powder
8-12 oz hot water

Add 1 tablespoon roasted carob powder for a richer drink – 72 calories
Add dates for sweetness, or cashews for a creamy drink.

Other hot beverage options

Try blending hot water with one or more of these options:

a banana
a small handful of dried mulberries
raisins
dried figs
dried apricots

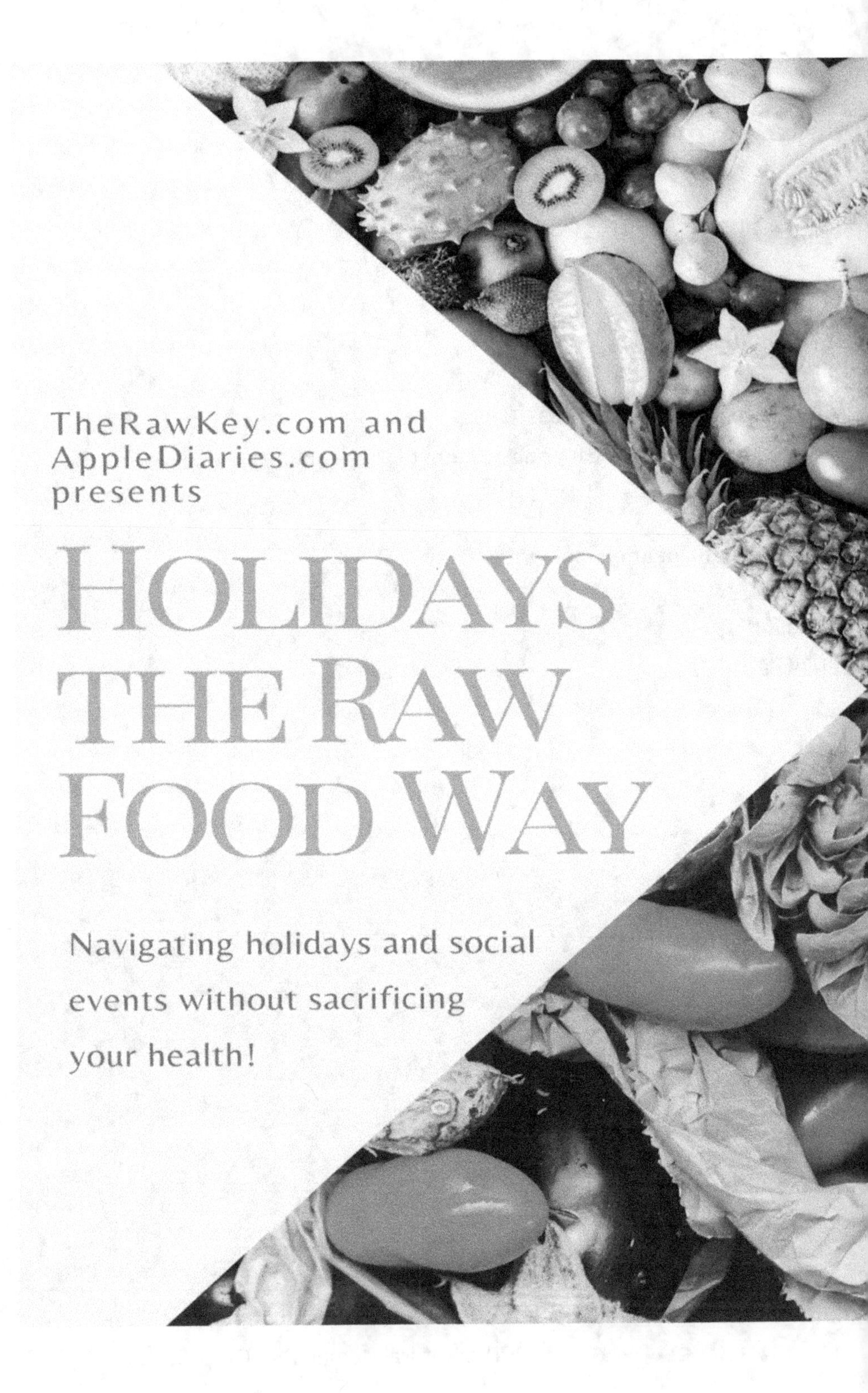

HOLIDAYS THE RAW FOOD WAY

Navigating holidays and social events without sacrificing your health!

Holiday Guide

Holidays and social gatherings can be difficult when we are transitioning back to the natural lifestyle. Here are some strategies to help you be able to enjoy these times without getting too far off track.

Coping Strategies from Lauren

Holidays, Gatherings and other Social Pressures

Approaching the end of the year brings some of the biggest eating and hedonism celebrations of the year with Thanksgiving here in America and Christmas just around the corner. I thought it might be nice to talk about some coping mechanisms to help handle these types of big events as well as the more mundane social gatherings like lunch or dinner with a friend.

I suppose there's no magic bullet to help us all navigate these situations, but I'll mention a few things that seem to have helped me cope.

- *Bring your own food, when possible*, be it a potluck situation or otherwise, it can really help. A nice salad, a ripe bunch of bananas, or a bag of grapes or apples can save us from nervous eating or overindulging in more harmful options. Even if the host is providing all the food. I would caution against going too far into the diet subject because most people take what they eat very personally. But you can merely say something like, "I have some dietary restrictions and I still wanted to come and participate and enjoy everyone's company."
- *At restaurants, order salads.* If you're going out to eat and feel compelled to order something, I've found most restaurants offer some type of salad that's minimally offensive. Usually called "garden salad" or "side salad" on the menu. Usually some type of vinaigrette dressing is a relatively safe option. Depending on the type of place you can often just ask for a simpler version of one of the other salads too.

- o *Take time for yourself.* I've also found that taking a quiet moment to remind myself before an outing or an event that the people are the real important part and not the food can be very helpful. If I'm really going out with people or celebrating a holiday more to socialize then this helps me de-emphasize the foods and enjoy the banter and social aspects more thoroughly.
- o *Fill up first.* Another tactic I often employ is to eat beforehand. If I fill up on ideal foods then even if I do waffle or indulge in some cooked or processed foods then I'm much more likely to indulge less. This will lead to less overall burden and a quicker recovery time.

Overall I've found these holidays, birthdays, and other gatherings can be a blessing because they've helped me realize and understand how much of an emotional endeavor eating truly is – at least for me, and I've heard these sentiments echoed by others many, many times. I've found that sometimes even if I do fill up on grapes or salad, I can find myself suddenly desperately searching for something to eat to help me deal with some sort of latent anxiety.

After going through this a few times I've been able to work through some of these issues. While it has become easier and easier to deal with these types of events, they're still not my favorite to participate in, so sometimes I will simply excuse myself if I feel overwhelmed. There's no sense in doing something you know will make you miserable just to try to fit in a little better.

Maria's Thoughts

Have you ever found yourself the focal point, or at the center of attention during a gathering because you were eating all the fruit and salad while everyone else was eating everything but?

Back when I first learned about the diet / disease connection, the information that I learned came so sudden and unexpectedly (I had to stop operations of an entire farm to change my diet/lifestyle), so I'll admit, I had trouble explaining to others what I had learned, and why I was doing what I was doing.

I experienced issues navigating dinner parties/gatherings because people would notice my new eating habits (which didn't sit well with them) and before I knew it, if I wasn't careful, the whole table would be focusing on me and my dietary choices.

It didn't help matters that I was quite passionate and upfront about the new information that I had learned. However, because I didn't yet possess good health myself, during those beginning couple of years, most of what I tried to explain to others fell on deaf ears, and the information that I was trying to share didn't flow properly.

Fast forward a few years, and I can say that I have learned a few important lessons on how to navigate these situations, and to not become the focal point, or center of attention when surrounded by mixed eaters (until we are ready and welcoming of a healthy debate).

#1 When preparing food, bring a dish for others to accompany that giant salad, or fruit plate you're bringing, such as a rice dish, potatoes, cooked vegetables, etc. You may not plan on eating it yourself, that is okay, the others will feel more at ease and won't feel the urge to attack, seeing you with all that food!

#2 Do not preach; do not bring up the topic of health and how unhealthy meat and animal products are unless someone else brings it up first.

#3 Load up your plate with what you want to eat and make no apologies – if someone asks, tell them you may dig into other foods after but right now you want a delicious salad!

#4 If someone asks you why you're not eating the other foods, explain briefly that you simply do not feel your best eating them. It's the long winded explanations that tend to grow into situations we didn't intend.

Seeing you doing things differently, others may feel the reflection, it's as if your healthier habits are reflecting, and causing them to examine their own habits – and most people do not want to think about their unhealthy choices, so they feel better about themselves if they attack or ridicule what you're doing instead.

It's nothing personal, it's a form of self-protection and old habit/tradition preservation. Not many people welcome change, and they will almost always take the path of least resistance. Little do they realize that their path of least resistance eventually builds up to higher levels of difficulty in their lives once their toxic accumulations overload the body.

We must be patient and kind no matter what situation we find ourselves in. The best course of action when dealing with people is to lead by example because people notice, and become curious, when someone breaks through societal programming and starts doing things differently. Let them approach you, until then, do your own thing.

True health is wealth! Health results from healthy living. When we live in health, we naturally live in the moment because pain is no longer the focal point.

Holiday Menu 1

4 Course Sit Down Dinner

Appetizer Course

Raw Stuffed Mushrooms

Soup & Salad Course

Creamy Tomato Soup

Kale & Brussels Sprout Salad with Lemon Mustard Dressing

Entree Course

Raw Holiday Loaf

Dessert Course

Raw Cheesecakes with Cranberry Jam

Recipes for Holiday Menu 1

Raw Stuffed Mushrooms

Full recipe 860 calories

If 2 servings 430 calories each, if 4 servings 215 calories each

1 box cremini mushrooms

2 tbsp Bragg Liquid Aminos *

Cashew Cream (Full recipe 375 calories)

½ cup cashews

juice of 1 small lemon

¼ cup water, or more to desired consistency

Pesto (Full recipe 420 calories)

2 cups baby spinach or baby kale

½ cup sunflower seeds

4-6 large basil leaves *

1 tsp lemon zest

juice of ½ a lemon

Clean mushrooms, remove the stems and discard or save for raw veggie burgers, place mushroom tops in a small container with Bragg Liquid Aminos, place lid on container and shake well to coat the mushrooms. Set aside to marinate, shaking the container every few minutes to distribute the Braggs.

Cashew Cream:

In a food processor or blender, combine the cashews, lemon juice and water and process until very smooth. Set aside.

Pesto:

In the food processor combine the baby spinach and/or baby kale, sunflower seeds, basil, lemon zest and lemon juice. Process until well combined but with a little texture.

Assembly:

Lay out mushrooms upside down on a serving tray. Taking a small spoon, scoop the pesto into the cavity in the mushroom. Evenly distribute pesto across all mushrooms. Then top with a dollop of cashew cream. Serve at room temperature, or dehydrate for 2-3 hours to warm.

Creamy Tomato Soup
630 calories

6 tomatoes
¼ cup tahini
5-6 sundried tomatoes
juice of 1 lemon
2 stalks celery
Optional: fresh basil *

Blend all ingredients until very smooth. Blend for 1-2 minutes for a warm soup. Optionally top with fine shredded basil as a garnish.

Kale & Brussels Sprout Salad with Lemon Mustard Dressing
415 calories

5-6 leaves kale, shredded
10 brussels sprouts, shredded
1 apple, shredded
½ head of green cabbage, shredded

Dressing:
2 tbsp mustard *
2 lemons, zested and squeezed
4-5 medjool dates

Blend all dressing ingredients, add water 1-2 tbsp at a time as needed to blend. (For a non-irritant option simply omit the mustard and add a little extra water)

Raw Holiday Loaf

1900 calories

Make in advance – Uses Dehydrator

Marinate First:
2 cups portobello or cremini mushrooms, roughly chopped
2 tbsp Bragg Liquid Aminos

Grind together first:
1 cup almonds
1 cup walnuts
¾ tsp dried thyme *
¼ tsp dried sage *
½ tsp onion powder *
½ tsp garlic powder *
¼ cup chopped parsley *

2 stalks celery, roughly chopped
¼ cup sundried tomatoes, soaked
4 dates, soaked
½ red bell pepper
1 tsp lemon juice

For the best flavor, marinate the mushrooms overnight in the Bragg Liquid Aminos. Grind the nuts and spices in a food processor until fine. Transfer to a bowl and set aside.

Place remaining ingredients in the food processor, including the mushrooms and process until it starts to stick together but there are still some medium fine chunks.

Pour into a bowl with the dry ingredients and knead until well combined. Shape into a rectangular loaf and place in the dehydrator for 8-12 hours.

Raw Cheesecake with Cranberry Jam

Full recipe 5600 calories

If 12 Servings 470 calories each, if 8 Servings 700 calories each

Crust:

1 cup pecans

1 cup dates

½ cup shredded raw coconut

Filling:

4 cups cashews, soaked 1-4 hours

⅓ cup coconut oil *

¾ cup lemon juice

¾ cup maple syrup *

1 tbsp vanilla extract *

water as needed to blend – about ¼ to ½ cup

Cranberry topping:

1 cup fresh cranberries

4 medjool dates, soaked 10-15 minutes

2-3 tbsp water

Crust: In a food processor combine all three ingredients and process on high until a ball begins to form. For a large cheesecake use a 9 inch springform pan. Press the crust into the pan and use a glass to press until it is even and sticking together well. If your mixture is too dry to stick together on its own add 1-2 additional dates or 1 tablespoon of water while the food processor is running.

For mini cheesecakes you will need a mini cheesecake pan or you could use a mini cupcake pan with cupcake liners and remove the liners before serving. This recipe makes about 30 mini cheesecakes. For the mini pans take about 1 tablespoon of crust mixture and press into the bottom of each hole.

Filling: Combine all ingredients in a blender or a food processor and blend until very smooth, adding water as needed to get it to a smooth creamy texture. You want to add as little water as possible so just add a little at a time.

Topping: Blend all ingredients until smooth. It should be a thick jam. If it is too thin add another date. If it is too thick to blend smoothly add a little more water.

Pour filling over the crust. Then using a spoon scoop about 1 tablespoon of jam on top of each mini cheesecake. If you are making a large cheesecake, place the cheesecake in the freezer for 1 hour before adding the jam so the cheesecake is firm and you can spread the jam. Freeze the cheesecakes for a few hours or until 1 hour before you are ready to serve. Keep in the fridge until you are ready to serve.

Holiday Menu 2

Buffet Style Holiday Meal

Appetizers

Simple Holiday Dip

Green Pea Dip

Zucchini Lasagna Bites

Desserts

Mulberry Apple Tarts

Raw Vegan Carrot Cake w/ Frosting

Raw Fudge Brownies

Recipes for Holiday Menu 2

Simple Holiday Dip

135 calories

2 tbsp of hemp seeds
1 cup peel zucchini

Blend hemp seeds and zucchini. Cut carrot, cucumber, bell pepper and celery to dip into this creamy sauce

Green Pea Dip

Full recipe 500 calories, 2 servings 250 calories per serving

1 cup green peas, fresh or frozen
½ cup raw almonds
juice of 1 lime
⅓ cup fresh cilantro * (optional)

Place almonds in a food processor and process until medium fine. Add remaining ingredients and process until smooth.

Zucchini Lasagna Bites
1260 calories

1-2 large zucchini

Cheese Layer
1 cup cashews, soaked 1-2 hours
juice of 1 lemon
water to blend

Tomato Sauce
4 medium vine ripe tomatoes
4-6 medjool dates
juice of 1 lemon
Optional add a sprinkle of basil *, oregano * and thyme * or some fresh basil *

This dish can be made in a small glass dish and then sliced into squares like sheet pan lasagna or made as an appetizer with individual rounds. In this instance we will be using the rounds for an appetizer but you can also do sheets by slicing the zucchini into long thin sheets about 1/8 inch thick. For our appetizer we will be slicing into ⅛ to ¼ inch thick circles. Place on a paper towel or clean dishcloth and set aside while you make the other elements.

Cheese Layer: Blend cashews and lemon juice with 1/3 cup water in a blender or food processor. Add additional water 1 tablespoon at a time until you reach a smooth but thick spreadable consistency.

Tomato Sauce: Blend all sauce ingredients until very smooth. The sauce should be thick, if it is too thin add 1 more date. The sauce will thicken slightly as the date absorbs more moisture.

Lay down a layer of zucchini sheets or circles. Top with cheese mixture, add another layer of zucchini, then another layer of cheese and another layer of zucchini. Top with tomato sauce.

Mulberry Apple Tarts

Full recipe 2050 calories, 30 tarts 68 calories each

Crust:
2 cups dates
2 cups dried mulberries
1 ½ cups shredded coconut
1 cup coconut flour

Filling:
1 gala apple
1 granny smith apple
1 fuji apple
2 honeycrisp apples
1 cup raisins
1 cup dates
juice of 1 lemon
2 tsp apple pie spice *

Topping:
¼ cup mulberries

Crust: Process all 4 ingredients in a food processor until they start to stick together. Press into mini cupcake pans (makes 30 small tarts) or 8" or 9" pie pan for a full-sized pie. Stick in the freezer to set while preparing other ingredients.

Filling: Set aside 1 honeycrisp apple and raisins. Combine the remaining filling ingredients in the food processor and process until you reach a chunky applesauce consistency. Take the remaining apple and finely chop it to roughly the same size as the raisins. Stir in raisins and chopped apples.

Fill crusts with filling and top with additional mulberries.

Raw Vegan Carrot Cake with Frosting (optional)

Full recipe 3200 calories

If 12 Servings 260 calories each, if 8 Servings 400 calories each

Carrot Cake (can be made into energy balls if no frosting is desired)

2 cups shredded carrot

2 cups of chopped / pitted medjool dates

2.5 cups chopped walnuts (optional)

1 tsp vanilla extract * (optional)

1-2 tsp cinnamon * (optional)

pinch of nutmeg * (optional)

½ cup of shredded coconut

¼ cup raisins

Stir together in a large bowl. Blend the dates in a little bit of water first until smooth / chunky, then add the rest of the ingredients and stir together.

Press all ingredients into a baking dish until compacted together. Top with raw cashew icing if desired or eat as is.

Raw Cashew Frosting

1 ¼ cup soaked raw cashews (drain)

½ cup water

2 tbsp of lemon juice

3 tbsp of maple syrup * (or homemade date syrup)

1 tsp vanilla extract * (optional)

Blend at high speed until creamy and thick. Spread on top of cake, refrigerate until hard and cut into squares and serve.

Raw Fudge Brownies

Full recipe 1420 calories

If 4 Servings 355 calories each, if 8 Servings 175 calories each

1 cup walnuts
1 cup dates
¼ cup raw cacao powder * (not hygienic) or ¼ cup raw carob powder (hygienic)

In a food processor, process walnuts until fine. Add cacao/carob and pulse until combined. Add dates and process until the dough ball forms. Form into a square about ½ inch thick. Slice into squares. Chill for 15-30 minutes before serving or serve at room temperature.

Holiday Menu 3

Classics Made Raw

Appetizer

Stuffed Mini Sweet Peppers

Entree

Zucchini Ravioli with Marinara Sauce

Side Dishes

Cauliflower Mash w/ Mushroom Gravy

Raw Stuffing

Cranberry Sauce

Dessert

Raw Pumpkin Pie

Recipes for Holiday Menu 3

Stuffed Mini Sweet Peppers

Full recipe 1080 calories, 4 servings 270 calories per serving

1 bag mini bell peppers

Stuffing

1 cup sunflower seeds, soaked 15 minutes to soften
1 red or orange bell pepper
2-3 sundried tomatoes, soaked for 15 minutes
juice of 1 lemon or lime

Strain sunflower seeds and sundried tomatoes but retain water from sundried tomatoes. Combine stuffing ingredients in a food processor. Process until fairly smooth or chunky, as you prefer. Add tomato soak water as needed to reach desired consistency. Slice peppers in half and remove seeds and stem. Lay on a serving platter and fill with sunflower spread.

Zucchini Ravioli with Marinara Sauce

Full recipe 1900 calories, 3 servings 633 calories per serving

The ravioli is prepared by using a vegetable peeler and peeling long strips of zucchini. To make a ravioli, criss-cross 2 strips with two strips making a "T".

Add a spoonful of filling and fold all four sides in to make a square little ravioli – repeat until all filling is used. Peel approximately 3 medium sized zucchinis (20 calories average zucchini).

Ravioli Filling (1610 calories)

1 ¼ cup soaked raw cashews (soak 1 hour)
¾ cup hemp seeds
¼ cup lemon juice
¼ cup water
1 tbsp of miso * (optional)

Once you've filled a small square baking dish with ravioli, add the raw marinara sauce (this sauce can be used on top of plain zucchini noodles as well).

Raw Marinara Sauce (230 calories)
1 pound tomatoes (roma, grape or cherry, on the vine, etc.), chopped
1 cup (3 oz) sun-dried tomatoes (not in oil)
1 teaspoon garlic powder *(optional)
2 tbsp shallots * (optional)
½ cup herbs * (cilantro, parsley or basil), medium packed (optional)

Soak sun dried tomatoes an hour prior and drain before using. Blend ingredients together until sauce-like consistency. Serve on top of zucchini noodles also!

Option – Hygienic Raw Sauce: (675 calories)
5-6 vine ripe tomatoes
4-5 sundried tomatoes
juice of 1 lemon
1 stalk of celery
5-6 medjool dates

Blend all ingredients until smooth.

Cauliflower Mash w/ Mushroom Gravy
Full recipe 1350 calories
4 servings 340 calories per serving

1 head cauliflower
½ cup pine nuts
1 cup cashews
2 tbsp white miso *
1 tsp garlic powder *
2 tbsp lemon juice or water

In a food processor combine all ingredients and process until smooth. Top with gravy – recipe next page.

Mushroom Gravy

1 8 oz container cremini mushrooms
2 tbsp Bragg Liquid Aminos *
1 tsp rubbed sage *
½ tsp thyme *
½ tsp rosemary *
¼-½ cup water

Combine ¼ cup water with remaining ingredients and blend until very smooth, thin to desired consistency with remaining water.

Raw Stuffing
650 calories

1 cup mushrooms
2 tbsp Bragg Liquid Aminos *
2 stalks celery
2 small carrots
½ cup pecans
2 dates
1 small head of cauliflower
½ tsp rosemary *
½ tsp sage *
½ tsp thyme *
¼ tsp nutmeg *

Marinate mushrooms in Bragg Liquid Aminos, set aside. In the food processor, process cauliflower until it is roughly the size of rice grains. Place in a medium sized bowl and set aside. Process pecans, dates, marinated mushrooms and spices until they form a thick paste. Stir together mushroom mixture with cauliflower until well combined. Process carrots until finely chopped. Hand chop celery into small pieces. Stir in carrots and celery. Serve at room temperature, or warm slightly in the dehydrator.

Raw Cranberry Sauce

680 calories

16 oz bag fresh cranberries

zest of 1 orange

½ cup orange juice (or more as desired for a thinner sauce)

1 cup dates – soaked in warm water for 10 minutes

Drain dates, combine all ingredients in a food processor, and process until chunky.

Raw Pumpkin Pie

Full recipe 2160 calories

If 12 Servings 180 calories each, if 8 Servings 270 calories each

Crust:

Combine equal parts:

1 cup almond flour

1 cup raw applesauce (purée a few dates with apples and a little lemon)

Mix together to form a crust – press into pie pan – let set in the refrigerator for at least an hour before filling.

Filling:

1¾ cup of raw pumpkin purée

¾ cup plant milk

4 dates

1 cup sweetener (date syrup, maple syrup *, etc.)

½ tsp cinnamon * (optional)

2 tsp allspice * (optional, can omit cinnamon if using allspice)

1 tsp vanilla extract * (optional)

¼ cup psyllium husk *

Blend everything together until smooth. Pour into pie crust and refrigerate until time to serve. Note: You can fill this crust with any raw, fruity filling such as apples tossed in date syrup & cinnamon (optional, not hygienic).

Summer Party Recipes

Date Strawberry Lemonade
340 calories

3 cups water
1 cup (140g) diced strawberries
¼ cup (50g) medjool dates (pitted and soaked in warm water for 10 minutes)
juice of 2 lemons (about 1/4 cup or to taste)

Combine all ingredients and blend until smooth. Add water if necessary.

Add more dates if you want sweeter lemonade. Add or substitute raspberries, blackberries, blueberries, or other fruit. Water content may need adjusted for plain lemonade without berries.

Raw Red Pepper Hummus
190 calories

2 red peppers, chopped
1 small zucchini, peeled and chopped
⅓ cup raw pumpkin seeds
1 tbsp fresh lemon juice
2 tsp onion powder * (optional)

Place all ingredients in a food processor, or a high-speed blender, blend on high until smooth. Add a little water at a time to make sure it is as thick or as thin as you want.

Bring this along with cut up veggies to ANY holiday party and I guarantee everyone will love it!!!

Hemp Seed Cream
135 calories

2 tbsp of hemp seeds
1 cup peeled Zucchini

Blend until smooth.

I Can't Believe It's Not Soy Sauce Dressing
110 calories

1 large tomato
1 oz of shelled tamarind
1 large stalk of celery
squeeze of lime juice

Blend until smooth.

Raw Kebabs

Note: This recipe can be raw or added to the BBQ for a transitional cooked version

You will need 10 bamboo kebab skewers for each type you plan to make, fruit or vegetable.

Fruit Kebabs (Full recipe 335 calories)
20 green or red grapes
1 chopped banana in pieces
10 chopped apple pieces
fresh pineapple chopped into pieces
10 pieces peeled mandarins or little oranges

This recipe is versatile and fun. You can use whatever fruit you have available, but for optimal digestion pay attention to food combining techniques. For guests, it's important that they enjoy the variety of fruit and see the vibrant colors.

Create melon skewers with cantaloupe, honeydew or other melons.

OR

Create acid fruit skewers with pineapple, oranges, kiwi and strawberries.

Use lemon juice to prevent the fruit skewers from oxidizing.

Fruit Skewer Date Dip (Full recipe 795 calories)
12 medjool dates (pitted and soaked)
touch of vanilla extract * (optional)

Blend the soft dates in a blender or food processor with a small amount of water that they were soaking in. Add a touch of vanilla, or use lemon instead. This dip is so simple and so sweet, it makes a nice addition for the sweet fruits such as banana and apple. Not recommended for melon skewers, eat melons alone!

Vegetable Kebabs (Full recipe 175 calories)

20 grape or cherry tomatoes
10 pitted green olives * or kalamata olives * (oil and garlic free preferably)
½ large sweet red or orange bell pepper cut into 10 slices
½ zucchini cut in 10 slices
½ cucumber cut in 10 slices
2 tbsp freshly squeezed lemon juice

Directions for Fruit and Vegetable Kebabs:

Thread ten 8 inch bamboo skewers each with one of each item, for example, 1 tomato, 1 pepper slice, 1 zucchini, 1 cucumber, and finish with a second tomato. Arrange the kebabs on a nice serving platter. Squeeze the lemon juice in a small bowl and brush each kebab with the lemon juice using a small pastry brush. Serve at room temperature or refrigerate 1-2 hours and serve chilled.

Carob Date Fudge Bites
Full recipe 1635 calories, 16 bars 102 calories each

2 cups tightly packed pitted medjool dates (soaked and drained)
1/4 cup warm water
1/2 cup coconut flour
1/4 cup coconut oil, melted *
1/3 cup carob powder

Add soaked dates and 1/4 cup warm water to food processor or blender. Blend until dates are finely chopped. Add coconut flour, melted coconut oil and carob powder to food processor and pulse until a sticky batter forms. Scrape / mix and blend again.

Transfer to 8" square baking dish lined with parchment paper and spread to an even layer. For a smoother top, add a sheet of parchment paper on top and smooth with a flat-bottomed object (like a drinking glass).

Transfer to the fridge to firm up for 30-60 minutes. Lift carob date bars out of the baking dish with the parchment paper. Slice into 16 bars and enjoy!

Camping Favorites – Dehydrator Recipes

Ratatouille

295 calories

4 tomatoes

1 eggplant, peeled

1 red pepper

1 yellow pepper

1 large or 2 small zucchini

Optional Seasonings (not hygienic – mild irritants): 1 tablespoon basil *, thyme *, rosemary *

In blender, combine 3 of 4 tomatoes with herbs and blend until smooth.

Dice eggplant into ¼ inch cubes and salt, set aside to drain.

Place blended mix on solid trays and dry until crumbly.

Cube remaining vegetables and combine with eggplant. Dry 12-24 hours, until crisp. Combine dehydrated ingredients. Use 1 cup water to 1 cup mix.

Chili

325 calories

4 tomatoes

1 tsp onion powder *

2 carrots, diced

1 cup of corn kernels

1 cup Mushrooms or 2 Portobellos

1 tbsp chili powder *

1 tbsp chipotle powder *

1 or 2 red, yellow or orange bell peppers *

salt, pepper *

Combine in a blender: onion powder, tomatoes, and spices and blend until smooth. Pour onto dehydration trays and dry until crumbly.

Dice carrots into ¼ to ½ inch cubes. Finely dice bell peppers. Combine with corn kernels and dry until crispy, 12-24 hours. Combine dehydrated ingredients. Use 1 cup water to 1 cup mix.

Corn Bark Stew

460 calories

1 cup peas
3-4 carrots, diced
2-3 celery stalks, diced
3 ears corn
1 tsp onion powder *
salt *, pepper *, cumin *, etc.

Blend corn with salt, pepper, and other seasonings. Dehydrate until crumbly, 12-24 hours.
Cube carrots, and celery into ¼ inch cubes and combine with peas.
Dehydrate 12-24 hours, until crispy. Combine dehydrated ingredients. Use 1 cup water to 1 cup mix.

Root Bark Stew

800 calories

2 tsp onion powder *
1 tbsp curry powder *
1 tbsp cumin *
3 large sweet potatoes *
½ pound parsnips *
½ pound carrots *
2-3 miscellaneous root veg (turnips, rutabaga, etc.) – *
2 tomatoes
3-4 stalks celery

In blender combine tomatoes, half celery, onion powder, curry powder, cumin, salt and pepper and any other seasoning, blend until smooth. Pour onto dehydrator trays, dehydrate until crispy.
Chop all root vegetables into ¼ to ½ inch cubes and dry until crispy, about 24 hours. Combine dehydrated ingredients. Use 1 cup water to 1 cup mix.

Sweet Potato Bark
345 calories

2 dry sweet potatoes *
½ cup apple juice
1 tbsp maple syrup *
1 tsp cinnamon *

Chop sweet potato into small chunks.
Place everything in blender and blend until smooth.
Pour onto dehydrator tray and dry until crispy.
Serve with oatmeal for breakfast or as dessert snack or side dish.

Monthly Support Group Information

Lauren Whiteman, Nat Farris and Maria Manazza, have been supporting and guiding others to build their health to optimal levels and heal their unwanted symptoms through the Natural Diet Support Group on Facebook each and every month without fail! As your group hosts, we share information that you aren't likely to hear in other health groups, and guide people on incorporating the information into their lives. We strive to provide the correct information needed to make wise choices about your health, so that you can get on with your life, do great things, and live up to your potential!

The goal of our Natural Diet Support Group is to teach sustainable habits and to help you transition at a pace that works for you. We teach step-by-step, day-by-day how to incorporate healthy habits and routines, and to bring the body back into health by eating in alignment with our natural diet. We focus on small changes and daily improvement so anyone can jump in right where they are and get started on improving their health right away. This group is for anyone who wants to eat more in alignment with their natural diet. It doesn't matter if you are already fully raw or still eating a SAD diet, we accept everyone and we are here to support you.

In addition to this Quick Start Guide, complete with Grocery Lists, Meal Plans, and over 100 Recipes, we also offer:

- Daily educational and motivational posts to make transitioning easier
- Check-ins and support from our 3 experts and other group members
- Your wellness questions answered by Lauren, Maria, and Nat
- A supportive group dynamic to cheer each other on and share helpful tips
- Tips for dealing with family, friends, and social situations
- Fasting tips and best practices
- How to deal with detox symptoms, and so much more!

If you are ready to build a pain free and joyous existence, and put in the daily effort, it isn't that difficult when you know what to do – which is where we come in!

We are here to help you to build those long lasting – sustainable healthy habits that serve the body to become healthy.

Our support group begins the first of each month, if you would like to join us, sign up at www.therawkey.com

"Nature does not hurry yet everything is accomplished" – Lao Tzu

Testimonials

The following are people's own words regarding their experience following the general recipes, diet, and principles outlined in this book. Some have been edited lightly for spelling or grammar but never for content.

- ➢ I've been on the Natural Diet for 6-7 weeks and my allergies nearly resolved in the first week, I was surprised. They were not fun! I also had crippling left knee pain from Fibromyalgia that has improved 90%. Still walking with a cane just in case it buckles too hard but I am almost ready to lose that as well. ~ Kevin

- ➢ My mom told me this morning that donuts don't taste good anymore! I believe all the fruits and salads I've been feeding her have changed her taste buds! And another thing...a small growth on my thigh has disappeared!! Hurray for Natural Hygiene!!! ~ Leyenda D

  - ➢ I took my blood pressure on January 1st this year. It was 153/104. I checked it today and it was 130/85! ~ Leyenda D

- ➢ The nerve pain in my feet has gone down a lot. The numbness is still there, but I'm sure that will heal too. I'm much more active because of it, I've started exercising again and I like going hiking more often... I'm happy. ~ Monika U

- ➢ I had a hole in my eardrum for many many years and now it's been confirmed by my doctor and audiologist that it's healed over. It was an OMG moment for me, I couldn't believe it , I've been on natural hygiene for about 3 months (not raw yet). Could my body have healed this in such a short time? I have no other explanation. I kept away from the antibiotics this time and let nature take its course. ~ Evelyn P

- ➢ Who knew the power of water?? I have a 'calcified' shoulder and some other medical term they use for it stemming from RA and possibly overuse of steroid injections into that area. It has limited movement (I couldn't swim anymore) but after drinking 2L of water daily for a month about 80% of my range of motion has returned! Think what I could achieve with 4 liters. But it [currently] takes me all day to drink 2 liters ~ Ina A

- ➤ BIG NEWS! BIG WIN! I know this group does not give much credence to blood tests. Understood. But I will take a moment to celebrate what looks like a win for me. More than 15 yrs ago I was diagnosed with hypothyroidism and eventually with an autoimmune disorder. My integrative doctor offered everything from armour thyroid to supplements, selenium, iodine, ashwagandha, curcumin. Nothing stopped the progression. Here is a rough breakdown of the TSH over the years:
  TSH
  2013 – 1.67
  2015 – 3.93
  2017 – 4.94
  2018 – 4.07
  2019 – 7.58
  Fall of 2020 started Dr. Morse protocol
  2021 (Jul) – 6.49
  Fall of 2022 transitioned to NH
  2023 (Feb) – 4.93
  2023 (Nov) – 4.43
  I think I stabilized my thyroid function thanks to NH! ~ Ina A

- ➤ Quick update from me if anyone is following along…. The cyst popped on Monday and is a few days from being healed completely! I'm incredibly grateful to Lauren, Maria and Nat and everyone else who has provided support and encouragement. It was really scary for me but I trusted my body and this lifestyle and it worked. Who would have thought hey, gosh what a crazy world we live in. I'm slowly unwinding all the programming. So yeah, just so so grateful ~ Sally

- ➤ My hot flashes are almost gone, I've lost 80 pounds. I haven't had my period in almost 4 years. I look younger and feel younger, I'm 53. I don't need anything but what I eat. ~ Mary F

- ➤ For the first time in my entire life, my digestive system is finally able to heal! It has been under constant attack and forced to perpetually work to repair itself over and over and over again... Even this last year that I have been raw I have not simplified enough to give my gut the break it needed! Thank you, Rachel V, for inspiring me to just eat bananas and lettuce. IT IS WORKING! I feel the repairing and rebuilding happening inside of me! It has been extremely uncomfortable this last week but I finally feel strength coming! And, because of all this healing, I had a tremendous appetite today! I ate TWO heads of iceberg lettuce after my morning coconut water, followed by 8 bananas and a plantain for lunch and later 6 bananas for dinner! What a miracle! I am so blessed to be here! Maria Manazza, Lauren Whiteman, Nat Farris – You are all a godsend and your wisdom, conviction and certainty help to anchor my faith in the process of the discomforts of healing. I can finally feel the turnaround of my body and I am rebuilding! Thank you for this amazing group and for all of you here, beyond words... Thank You! I am forever grateful for this community. ~ Kari W

- Last month I started increasing my water intake, fasting until 11 or 12 & saving my fat intake until evening & avoiding stimulants & irritants as much as possible. This month I have just experienced such a delightful menstrual period. No pain, no cravings, no blood (just a tiny amount of colour change). I've been high raw for 1 year and fully raw for almost 6 months of that. The only time I've experienced a period similar was when I was doing a sweet juicy fruit only challenge for a month that was impossible & miserable for me to stick to long term. Natural hygiene however is easy and a joy. Feeling so happy to no longer have to dread the challenging monthly period that would go on for a good 5 days. ~ Caro W

  - Put my kettle in storage today. Yay I'm completely off coffee, coffee substitutes & tea. Lauren Whiteman & Maria Manazza have been the hugest sources of information, inspiration & support on their raw hygienic challenge so far this month. And it's been great having my accountability buddy Gia K join me for it! Got me reconsidering so many things & with knowledge comes power to just say no to things that don't serve the body. Their information & dedication is exactly what I was needing. ~ Caro W

- So I've been eating raw since the March challenge and I can honestly say my mental health has improved 100%. I'm amazed at how much it's improved. It's absolutely incredible. I've suffered with depression, anxiety etc., since a child and I've had a lot of trauma over years and I've been trying so hard the last 3 years to deal with past traumas and heal relationships with family members but I've just felt so stuck. I've felt a lot of anger. I've had so much I've wanted to start achieving in my life but just have felt so overwhelmed with doing any of it that I was stuck in the same patterns and not moving anywhere. Since being raw, for the first time in my life my mind is so clear, it's never been so clear. My memory has improved. I've started reading, socializing, learning guitar, growing some food and working on projects I've been putting off. My anxiety has reduced 100% and I just feel so calm in every area of my life. My family has seen a massive change in me and they just can't believe the effects this way of living is having on me. I'm only at the beginning of my raw and healing journey and I don't eat perfectly and I still have my ups and downs and work to do but they are not so intense and overwhelming anymore and I feel I can deal with things in a much healthier way. I couldn't be happier about this. I just wanted to share this with everyone in hope it helps anyone. I've seen such changes in such a small amount of time. I Just feel so blessed that I've found this way of life and the truth and found this support group as it's been everything to me so thank you to the admins and of course everyone participating. ~ Cassie S

➢ I have been loosely following tenets of Natural Hygiene for almost 3 years; mainly the diet, many months strict, many months loose. This month I incorporated them all, and the effects are pretty dramatic. I am having feelings of vibrant health like I haven't had since I was a teenager. I am sleeping like a rock (on my active days). I cannot sit still again. I am talking to more people. I am hyper-motivated and spend a great deal of time thinking how much I appreciate everything and what I want to do for the future. A few other TMI improvements as well but I'll keep it at that. One takeaway I'd like to press on for others in this group is that even when you think you know it all, it is good to circle back from time to time with your mentors to see if you're leaving anything out. There is additional motivation as well! ~ Drew W

➢ Since I read the post on water I've been drinking a gallon+ a day. It has had a noticeable impact on cravings. I'm eating less both in the day and evening, I'd say by 15-25% as a whole, and not going to bed hungry either! Finally seeing some good movement on the scale as well. I think being dehydrated was bringing on craving-like feelings. Gallon+ a day is the new normal. ~ Drew W

➢ Another small success story! Every 2 to 3 months I have to get my bloods taken (Rheumatoid Arthritis) and usually my neutrophils and WBC are low but this time they are classed as normal, first time in about 5 years.
~ Helen A

➤ Since incorporating the Natural Hygienic diet/lifestyle I no longer have asthma! Weight loss was needed, I'm also happier, more energetic and self-confident. Additionally, I'm sleeping better and have softer skin too!
  ~ Bethany L

➤ I feel generally lighter and less heavy inside my body. My skin is clear, my anxiety has lowered significantly, and my ability to manage stress is at an all time high. I have more energy than I can ever remember having in life. I'm a single mom and sometimes only get 3-4 hours of sleep but still make it through every day without crashing mid-day. With our move, I work on packing, cleaning, and sorting for 12 hours a day and have the stamina and strength to get through it! I've also found I am significantly more in tune with my body. I can tell if a healing event is going to start and can immediately begin fasting. I can also detect when I've come into contact with a toxin or non ideal ingredient because my body gives me cues like lethargy, a headache, increased thirst, or digestive discomfort. I started this journey just to try it out and here I am almost 15 months later still trying it out. I have also felt freer with my food choices. I can go anywhere at any time because I can always bring my food with me! Grocery shopping is a breeze because I get the same things every time with the occasional variation if I'm trying a new recipe. Overall, I feel like I am the healthiest I've ever been. ~ Lesli C

➤ I have just picked up my blood results (I know, I know) and I can't believe what I'm seeing! A little background: I'd become anemic in September 2006 (nearly 17 years ago) as a result of cesarean and never really recovered from it. My body wouldn't tolerate iron supplements so I started seeing naturopathic doctor over 3 years ago. They put me on lactoferrin, colostrum, copper, some probiotics supporting iron absorption. I felt better and more functional but when I tried to live without those last year I become very much nonfunctional within 2 months. I thought I'm destined to be dependent on them for the rest of my life. I went hygienic on 22nd May this year and ditched all my supplements. Part of me wanted to have hope and the other part honestly feared that I'm going to die within weeks. I stopped having any symptoms of anemia within 2 weeks of being on the diet. Going back to my blood test. I AM NOT ANEMIC!!! Not only that – all my blood cells are of a normal shape (my hemoglobin would fluctuate in and out of range for years but even when it was borderline within range, blood cells were odd shape and 'nonfunctional' and I would have problems

breathing). Looking at my B12 – the value has doubled (from mid-range to the top range). My ferritin and iron are still below range BUT are higher than when I was on supplements. Don't let anyone tell you this diet will starve you – it'll heal you! PS. I know we shouldn't keep checking blood as it changes from moment to moment, but I wanted/needed some sort of reassurance and confirmation. I can also use it to show to people who challenge me saying natural hygiene is a diet of starvation and that you cannot survive without supplements (I do struggle sometimes when discussing what I eat now, especially with family – now I don't have to).
~ Gosia A

> I saw a post in the Terrain group about herbs and reading the responses of some people had me thinking so much about how horrendously brainwashed we all have been. It's so weighty for me to see that so many people just can't see this common sense information. I was visiting a naturopath for years in the past and I did so much supplements and herbs and I did not experience any healing. Then I did so many Dr Morse herbs and each time my body reacted so violently to all these herbs. One day I saw a post by Maria where she was addressing this issue on herbs. I remember telling my husband about it and I remember telling him at that time I think I agree with her, this make so much sense, but at that time I was so afraid I think to let go because we have this horrible idea ingrained in us that we need something from outside to fix our body...that's how we grew up thinking that we need a magic pill, herb, supplement because we don't have a CLUE how the body works and what the body is capable of. Then I started to follow this woman that by eating a raw food diet save herself from having surgery to remove 6 fibroids and her uterus and the first thing she said is that she did not consume any other thing other than living foods, and then another one that was sick almost all of her life and in one year and a half of eating raw foods no herbs she is completely a different human being. Then when I started the challenges back in November I was ready, I stopped every herb that I was taking that by that time were very minimal... I have to say that for the first time in 3 years of experiencing the most horrendous severe inflammation (liquid retention in my belly) every month in my ovulation this last 2 cycles I have seen a little bit of improvement. I have a long way to go I know, but even though I haven't seen major changes yet, in the past I felt that I was getting worst each time, now even though I can't really explain it or put it in words is like

I feel there is something good happening in the right direction little by little. Hope everyone is doing good! ~ Jessica M

> Before starting all this journey with my health in 2020 I was an active person doing exercise or a sport. I will go to the gym to exercise, nothing excessive, but active. I also was either doing cycling, (my favorite), walking or jogging, etc. When I started to experience all the inflammation that I go thru and also doing some things that made my situation worst (using natural medicine like supplements and herbs and other therapies like coffee enemas) I started to feel that I was getting worse and worse and so weak. I was having numbness in my right leg, discomfort in my spine, tingling on my right shoulder and a lot of muscle soreness. This went on and I stop doing exercise since 2021. Then I started to eat all raw and I was feeling at times even more weak. At times I was concerned about not doing any type of light exercise because I consider that have been so long, but I really felt that I couldn't. Until now... I am starting to feel so much better. I have a stationary cycling bike and today I just sat on it and I thought oh my goodness I actually feel that I can do this again. I am starting to feel stronger, I also notice that my hair is getting more abundant and I don't notice too much hair falling at all. I also notice that the discomfort that I was experiencing in my spine is basically not there, the tingling I don't know the last time I felt it and the numbness on my right leg is so much less, seriously our bodies are amazing. ~ Jessica M

> Before I found this group, I did a parasite cleanse and series of colonic irrigation. One a week for 6 weeks. All very harsh on my system. I always had trouble with constipation. After changing to the natural hygiene diet, I have no trouble going and my digestion is functioning so well. ~ Nicole C

> Just wanted to share a quick update about what I am going through since I've been doing raw for 16.5 months. For about the first 14 months, I was only doing fruits (no greens) and avoiding water because I was told we should only derive our water from fruit. Life for the first year or so:

* Felt great all summer, detox symptoms off and on to the point I couldn't even walk very far.
* By September last year, my legs were burning with dryness as usual for me, that time of year – had to use something topical to relieve it, which I later realized wasn't recommended.

* I craved sweet fruits like dates and figs but would get very dry if I ate them. Seems like Fall weather I always need more sweet in my life to warm me up and keep up with the generally active nature of the season.

* By Fall, I started taking interest in some cooked food with Fall flavors. The craving grew and I was indulging regularly (and feeling horrible after it) – sometime 3-4 times a week.

* The indulgence carried on through winter although I was getting tired of it but I couldn't stand the cold with what I was eating otherwise, cooked food seemed to keep me warm (acids burning from inside for warmth?).

* My dental health wasn't that great but that was explained as acids leaching out into the mouth from detoxing sinuses and need to be rinsed off often throughout the day, made sense but doing that didn't help a whole lot.

* Oh, and I was on a protocol for several months that included 7 or 8 of Dr Morse's herbs.

Life since introduction of greens and 1 gallon water in late July:

* I used to drink 1-1.5 gallons when eating cooked but the 14 months of starving myself for water, I had to start with only a quart a day – couldn't drink any more than that. I was able to work up to a gallon in a month – now I can drink up to 1.5 gallons sometimes, no forcing, but definitely try to hit at least a gallon every day.

* With greens, especially, my dental health improved to the point I no longer felt the need to brush my teeth and haven't since then. I do rinse my mouth morning and night and brush occasionally when I eat fats and have something sticking to my teeth or just want my mouth to feel fresh.

* My legs got dry a bit and were burning mid-Sept but that went away and I did nothing to relieve it other than scratch a bit. My legs still look dry but don't itch or burn anymore.

* With water regimen, I started waking up to pee 3 times every night – around 12:30 - 2:30 and 4:30 which would vary by +-30 minutes. Now, I wake up only twice within the assimilation cycle (before 4 am)

* No more cravings for cooked food! I think hydration and minerals from greens is what I needed. Now I can enjoy dates and figs every day and nuts every other day or so. BTW, you don't eat nuts in Dr Morse's world.

* I am maintaining my weight at 120 lbs. (I could gain some). Looking forward to longer fasts to clean out my malabsorption.

* I quit taking Dr M herbs when I learned from NH that herbs are harmful and a burden to the body, which matched my own experience. Now, I feel my body is healing more efficiently than ever since it has nothing burdening it and interfering with its innate wisdom.

* Overall, I feel more grounded, have the best mental clarity I've ever had which has greatly improved my work performance, especially decision-making (I am highly self-critical and have very high standards).

So, I am sooooo grateful for the little shifts I learned to make from NH, it's turned my life around for the better. Now, I just need to figure out how to get my girls to do what I do to feel better, both physically and mentally.

~ Vaibhav B

➢ My 3+ year old has been daytime toilet trained for about 8 months – it was so slow going for her. But night time has been back and forth with her being able to keep it dry or not. I started about 2 months ago with myself eating a ton more fruit and salads and more and my family is joining in. It's now been 2 weeks of my 3 year old having zero wet diapers at night! You guys I 100% believe it was from incorporating more fruit and veg – we are for sure still transitioning but I think it was too much burden for her kidneys before with all the butter and meat and milk and cheese we were doing – we are not 100% done with all those but we have not done meat in several weeks and we went from drinking 5 gallons of raw milk a week to zero! So a massive reduction in several areas plus adding in all the good stuff! This is so exciting! Also my baby stopped having 99% of his reflux issues when I switched my diet imperfectly over! My husband shared a win today – he has not had reflux the past couple months since he switched to vegan and more raw foods. And at this point he has eaten more lettuce in the last couple months than he did in his whole life combined I'm sure! Maybe several times over. So proud of him!!"

~ Hildegard B

➢ So as we are at the 2 week end I want to share my wins and my goals for the final 2 weeks; firstly however I want to spread some appreciation and gratitude to this wonderful group and how supportive you all are. And to any lurkers who are watching quietly from behind the scenes not feeling it to post...I used to be you! But this time round I have posted and doing so and the received support is a terrific boost to help fulfil your goals. I also want to appreciate Maria Manazza, Nat Farris and Lauren Whiteman without whom I couldn't have got this far! So to the wins and goals:

Wins

* drinking without fail 3L of water daily – WITHOUT any squash just straight water

* I have gone from 18st 3lbs to 17st 2lbs – long way to go to be well and healthy but it's a good start

* no acid reflux what so ever and not bought any antacid remedy in 12 days
* now sleeping for at least 5 hours solid whereas previously to this I would wake up every 2 hours for a pee, now realize my bladder was so irritated by the acids
* managing 2/3rds of a head of lettuce everyday still with shop bought dressing and lots of fruit but only bananas, oranges, grapes
* got a distiller and dehydrator and NH book
* fallen of the wagon 3 times but got straight back on and didn't allow it to destroy the bigger picture
GOALS FOR NEXT TWO WEEKS
* increase water to 4L by end of support group
* actually use distiller and dehydrator and read the book
* try more varieties of fruit
* eat whole head of lettuce
* make better choices if falling off the wagon or grip on a little tighter so I don't fall would be even better
* rest more and let body do its thing
We are all where we need to be lots of love to you all ~ Emma H

➤ Hello!..I'm so happy to be here again for my 3rd month after following Terrain group for a bit longer. My first meal today at noon – 3 apples and 1 mango with greens. I've had 2 Liters H20 today already which is big for me. I have difficulty breathing so pausing to swallow can be challenging...I found straws to be better with water so that helps a lot! I'm here to help gain weight, improve breathing, dental caries, strength, and digestion. I was high raw mostly fruit and the above things were pretty bad. I have significantly increased my greens and found that to be a total game changer. Also more focus on simpler ingredients and food combining. I have already noticed my one tooth is remineralizing, better digestion, more energy, and weight has stabilized. Lots of game changing tips like "do nothing" and rest. Like the last time I got sick..no herbs, no meds, just hydrate, hydrate, hydrate and rest and let the body do its things. Very grateful for Lauren Whiteman Nat Farris and Maria Manazza and this group. I enjoy learning from everyone and inspired by your pics. ~ Nina G

➤ I wanted to share a success story. I had my last ever filling today at the biological dentist with no anesthesia and I didn't feel a thing. I think since eating this way my pain levels have completely shifted. I have been very sensitive my entire life but my body seems to thrive this way as in I'm in my natural habitat even if I cut myself or bruise myself it heals and clears up during the day and I don't feel pain. I know some people tend to feel everything eating this way but I am the reverse seeing as I felt my entire life, plus my metabolism is at its optimal, not only that I rest my body more often and have naps and if I fall off the bandwagon I get no symptoms. My body flushes it right out naturally. ~ Ana G

➢ I thought I'd share a small win or bit of progress I've made after about 2 months of eating hygienically and drinking a gallon of water a day. I can't remember the last time my nails were able to grow this long without cracking and breaking. I know it's a bit superficial, and that most of us have real health problems, but it's pleasing to me nonetheless, and I think it is a sign of the internal progress my body has made. My teeth are also doing better – they are less sensitive and I am able to brush more thoroughly so they look cleaner. I attribute this to my increase in consumption of greens and water for sure. I was eating a fruitarian diet last year that didn't incorporate very many greens and barely any water and was experiencing a ton of dental issues. ~ Lura D

➢ Changes notes after initial 40 days of strict NH (including roasted peanut butter)
  * Days 3-35 I had constant thick yellow mucus, even lost my taste and smell for a week.
  * Had 2 periods on days which were lighter than usual and also found didn't get constipated for those days.
  * Days 20-27 I did a 7-day water fast as developed tonsilitis symptoms. Day 26 felt better, then just mild sore throat til day 32.
  * Had had thrush coming and going with my cycle for the best part of the previous year. This seemed to improve a little then got to the worst it's ever been around day 15. Felt much better by day 22 and fully gone by day 31.
  * On day 26 I realized my weak left wrist seemed to have healed?! For a few years I couldn't put pressure on my left wrist in the press-up position – it would go weak and then feel achy for a week afterwards if I did. Don't remember injuring it but maybe I did. Now it feels the same strength as the right one and no pain! ~ Jodie L

  ➢ This was in April-May. Left wrist still normal (in September). Thrush returned in June when I fell off the wagon for a few weeks, but went away again once I started eating NH again (and has stayed away despite not being as strict). Periods have remained at 2 heavy days instead of 3. ~ Jodie L

- Progress Report: I'm a month in…definitely not perfect, but I'm glad to report that my cravings are starting to diminish. My son's reflux has nearly disappeared. When I deviate, even with red onion or cilantro, he spits up. I can't express the gratitude I have for finding answers to my son's source of pain. I have so much more energy. I am so thankful to feel a renewed sense of zest for living. And to feel like I can play and keep up with my toddler. My PPD has really turned around. I went through a pretty tumultuous emotional detox. I'm kind of scared to jinx myself, but I'll just say I'm feeling pretty good these days. Thank you to the group leaders who are educating the public and evangelizing this way of life. I'm forever grateful. ~ Carissa LW

- The support, guidance and kindness that I have received within this support group has been incomparable to anything else. I entered this support group battling a severe illness and today, almost 8 months later working within this group, my health has returned and skyrocketed. I have become very inspired, and will forever continue within this incredible group. The 3 leads of this group, Lauren Whiteman, Nat Farris and Maria Manazza are exceptional guides, highly knowledgeable and devoted. The group feels like a family and has gifted me so much. ~ Anonymous

Have you experienced improvements after switching
to the natural human diet?
Do you have a success story you'd like to share?
Visit www.therawkey.com to submit via our testimonials page,
and maybe you'll see your story in our next book.

Meet your Moderators
Lauren Whiteman

Lauren has been studying health and wellness for over twenty three years. She studied and followed all of the mainstream health advice, searching for answers and cures to her chronic health conditions, but kept getting more sick, doing all of the things we are told are healthy for us – vegetarian since age 11, no fast foods, soda, junk food, etc. She was eating a diet of predominantly whole foods, lots of whole wheat/grains, cooked 95% of food at home, and still was not finding relief. She suffered from chronic pain, chronic fatigue, IBS, a golf ball-sized mass in her breast, acne, suicidal depression, insomnia, migraines, anxiety, was 70 pounds overweight and miserable.

So she dug deeper and started making other changes. She removed cheese and eggs and became vegan at the age of 26 after watching a documentary about the dairy industry, and then began to transition to a raw diet at age 30.

First trying "Raw till 4", then going high raw/high fat raw, and then moving to a fruit centered diet over about 2 years. Once she moved to High Fruits/Terrain Model – the natural human diet; it took about 18 months to heal completely of ALL OF her prior health ailments. Many of her symptoms began to subside on high fat raw but moving to the natural human diet is where she saw the greatest gains.

In addition to hosting the monthly Natural Diet Support Group, Lauren is a moderator of the Terrain Model Refutes Germ Theory group on Facebook as well as the author of TheRawKey.com website, where she provides valuable information about natural hygiene and the natural human diet.

Lauren also runs a group for cats and dogs on Facebook called Natural Dog & Cat Diet Group with TheRawKey.com teaching people how to feed their pets of their own natural diet, and return them to health and vitality, extending their lives. She also rescues senior dogs and other animals who are given a death sentence by veterinarians, and by simply feeding them the way they are designed to eat, conditions are reversed, and happy, healthy animals emerge from hopelessness.

Maria Manazza

Maria's health issues began when she was young, from the age of six she suffered excruciating leg pain which doctors could not figure out. Her childhood was affected by the constant pain and everything that goes with it. As a young adult she was prescribed pain medications and sleeping pills, even birth control pills (in case it was hormonal) and told that it probably would not go away. A nerve specialist told her that she should get used to pain medication for a lifetime because there was no solution as she was diagnosed with a dead nerve in her leg.

Maria also experienced a vaccine reaction at the age of 16. After a Hepatitis B vaccine, she blacked out and suffered with temporary paralysis, she had to lay down for a few hours until she could see, hear and walk again. Looking back, she thinks this is when her eyesight began to decline. She lost motivation and concentration which affected her life, socially and academically.

At the age of 35, she had moved to a 7-acre organic farm. They had grass fed cows, chickens, organic eggs and raw milk. They believed the food produced from their land to be the healthiest food available and she was expecting to heal her symptoms. But her condition continued to decline, migraine headaches, cysts, acne , chronic fatigue, body pain, rashes, insomnia, and other symptoms became increasingly worse and she experienced hopeless depression. One day, sitting on the couch many years ago at the farm, she suddenly couldn't stand up. She had lost control of her muscles and her whole body hurt. It was after this incident that she began questioning her organic farm diet that she believed was the healthiest available. Reading "The PH Miracle" by Dr. Young revealed to her that meat, dairy and eggs should be eliminated from the human diet as they are acidic foods, which she did immediately. She slowly began to feel symptom relief. A short time later they moved from the farm, as it became a fruitless and harmful endeavor.

After reading Arnold Ehret's book "Rational Fasting," she incorporated the mucusless diet, fasting and intermittent fasting into her routine which brought her even closer to health. Then reading Dr. Robert Morse's information years later she began to develop a deeper understanding of the detoxification process the body must go through. Maria began studying the works of Herbert Shelton and

TC Fry after joining the Terrain Model Refutes Germ Theory group and became a moderator soon after, working alongside Lauren Whiteman, Nat Farris and other dedicated knowledgeable moderators while incorporating natural hygiene principles. Living on the natural diet, Maria no longer suffers with symptoms such as daily or weekly migraines, chronic fatigue, nail biting, cysts, skin rashes, age spots, itchy scalp, acne, skin tags, varicose veins, alcoholism, anger, anxiety, nervousness, and more.

Today she lives symptom free and helps moderate the Natural Diet Support Group with Lauren Whiteman and Nat Farris. The support group starts the first of each month and teaches how to properly transition to a health promoting natural diet while maintaining sustainable healthy habits, in order to help people heal their symptoms and disease issues.

Nat Farris

Nat Farris experienced many health conditions from a young age such as chronic ear infections, hypothyroidism, ADD symptoms, and allergies which over time morphed into chronic pain and fibromyalgia, leading him to drop out of school and eventually become bedridden for a stretch in his late 20s and early 30s.

He was able to completely relieve or greatly reduce all symptoms by following the principles of natural hygiene and water fasting and now enjoys helping others through the process of taking responsibility for their health and bettering themselves through change in diet and lifestyle habits.

Among the issues Nat that has addressed and healed from are fibromyalgia, chronic pain issues, ADD, chronic neck issues from birth trauma, sciatica, spinal stenosis, hip issues from a congenital birth defect, sleep issues, bloating, obesity (lost about 150 lbs.), and hypothyroidism.

The resident expert in fasting, Nat hosts the Natural Diet Support Group each month with Lauren and Maria, in addition to moderating the Terrain Model Refutes Germ Theory Group on Facebook with them.

The Natural Human Diet Quick Start Guide

A Companion to The Raw Key's

Natural Diet Support Group

TRANSITION BACK TO

THE NATURAL HUMAN DIET

WITH EASE

Updated to include even more information on how to transition to the natural human diet, with additional meal plans and recipes, including Summer Party Recipes and Camping Favorites; information about our monthly support group – The Natural Diet Support Group on Facebook, and testimonials from group members.

TheRawKey.com

AppleDiaries.com

Revision 2.22
February 2025

www.ingramcontent.com/pod-product-compliance
Lightning Source LLC
Chambersburg PA
CBHW071015250726
48653CB00005B/1621